THE MAKINGS OF A MODERN EPIDEMIC

The Makings of a
Modern Epidemic
Endometriosis, Gender and Politics

KATE SEEAR
Curtin University, Australia

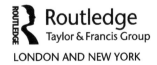

LONDON AND NEW YORK

First published 2014 by Ashgate Publishing

2 Park Square, Milton Park, Abingdon, Oxfordshire OX14 4RN
52 Vanderbilt Avenue, New York, NY 10017

Routledge is an imprint of the Taylor & Francis Group, an informa business

First issued in paperback 2018

British Library Cataloguing in Publication Data
A catalogue record for this book is available from the British Library.

The Library of Congress has cataloged the printed edition as follows:
Seear, Kate, author.
  The makings of a modern epidemic : endometriosis, gender and politics / by Kate Seear.
    pages cm
  Includes bibliographical references and index.
  ISBN 978-1-4094-6082-4 (hardback) 1. Endometriosis. 2. Women's health services.
3. Women--Health and hygiene. I. Title.
  RG483.E53S44 2014
  618.1'42--dc23

                                                                2013034127

ISBN 978-1-4094-6082-4 (hbk)
ISBN 978-0-367-07802-7 (pbk)

Contents

Acknowledgements

Although it is now a very different beast, this book originated as a PhD in sociology that was supported by an Australian Postgraduate Award (APA). I would like to thank both the School of Political and Social Inquiry and the Department of Sociology at Monash University for their administrative and financial support for the initial project. This book would not have been possible without, first and foremost, the generosity and spirit of 20 women with endometriosis who agreed to be interviewed for this study. I am tremendously indebted to all of them for their time, and for the stories they shared. I also wish to thank those who assisted me to locate participants for the study, including friends and family, and staff and volunteers from the Endometriosis Association of Victoria.

I am also indebted to my supervisors who were a wonderful support throughout my candidature. This journey started in 2003, with Jan van Bommel, my Honours supervisor. Jan supported my decision to pursue a doctorate and guided me through the first two years of candidature, forever instilling in me a love of feminist theory and practice. I owe an enormous debt of gratitude to Andrew Singleton, especially, who was my main supervisor throughout the candidacy. Andrew's patience, support, insight and enthusiasm sustained me throughout the many trials and tribulations of the project, as did our endless discussions about Australian cricket and the wonders of the Hawthorn Football Club.

I would also like to thank a number of people who have been important to me in various ways – first through my PhD – and later, in the writing of this book. I am grateful to Nick Economou, Narelle Miragliotta, Mark Davis, Steven Angelides, Michael Janover, Celia Roberts, Gayle Letherby, Anna Harris, Rebecca Conning, Daniel Edwards, Genevieve Heard, Claire Tanner, Ibrahim Abraham, Liudmila Kirpitchenko, Narelle Warren, Jennifer Sinclair, Jennifer Mitchell, Jenny Williams and Sue Stevenson. To my dear friends Marina Cominos, Zareh Ghazarian and Ben Whiteley – who put up with discussions about endometriosis over many years – thank you. I am also thankful to Alan Petersen for his guidance, wisdom, friendship and support. I am extremely grateful to Suzanne Fraser for her thoughts and comments on an early draft of this manuscript, her encouragement to write this book, and for her enthusiasm, sense of humour and friendship. Thanks, also, to the very talented British artist Kaye Sedgwick (http://www.kayesedgwick. co.uk/) who graciously provided the cover art for this book, and who shares my commitment to raising awareness about endometriosis.

Portions of this book have been previously published. Material in Chapter 3 appeared as 'Standing up to the Beast: Contradictory notions of control, un/

certainty and risk in the endometriosis self–help literature' in *Critical Public Health* (Seear 2009a). A component of the argument from Chapter 4 appears in *Health, Risk and Society* as '"Nobody really knows what it is or how to treat it": Why women with endometriosis do not comply with healthcare advice' (Seear 2009d). These materials have been reproduced with permission of the publishers.

I wish to thank my family, as well as the Dugmores, and all of my friends, including Lys, Dids, Meg and Ro, especially. I am particularly grateful to my sister Claire Seear, who has now put up with me for two books. And most of all, to Stewart Dugmore, who planted the seed that has grown into this book, and whose unending support and encouragement helped make it happen.

Finally, to my friend Lynette Watson, who continues to be an inspiration, and who reminds me every day why this book is needed.

Introduction:
Towards Pastiche

What is Endometriosis?

In 2005, I sat down to conduct the first of many interviews for a doctoral thesis exploring the experiences of women suffering from a chronic gynaecological disease known as endometriosis. Wanda, my first interviewee, was 26 years of age, and had suffered from the disease since she was a teenager. Over the course of two hours, she talked me through the onset of symptoms, her journey towards a diagnosis, and the repeated surgeries (six, at that stage) that she had undergone: first, to diagnose the condition and later, as a form of treatment. In the year leading up to our interview, Wanda's health had declined to such an extent that she had been formally certified as unfit for work – or medically 'disabled', to be more precise. Having obtained that certification, Wanda was now receiving financial support from the government in the form of a modest disability pension. Wanda's experience of endometriosis was similar, in many ways, to the experiences of other women that I would go on to interview for my study. Endometriosis had had a profound and significant effect on her life, a life that had come to be characterised by encounters with gynaecologists, bowel surgeons, urologists and naturopaths, and by cycles of invasive medical treatment.

Towards the end of our interview, however, something unexpected happened. Wanda nervously wondered if she might ask me a question. Confessing, with some embarrassment, that she still didn't really know *what endometriosis was*, Wanda asked if I wouldn't mind explaining the disease to her. Wanda's request both surprised and worried me. How could she not know what endometriosis was? How had the disease been explained to her in the past? What had her treating doctors been telling (or perhaps *not* telling) her? What was it like to live with this uncertainty, confusion and lack of clarity? How might this shape her lived experience of the disease? Inspired by my own encounters with feminist literature on the importance of open, two-way communications in the research encounter,[1] I quickly began a lengthy explanation of the condition as I understood it. Drawing upon my own experiences with endometriosis and all that I knew from medical texts, self-help books and other resources, I explained how and when the disease

---

1 There is now an enormous body of literature dealing with traditional forms of interviewing, feminist critiques of the interview and research method, much of which is formed through feminist explorations of empiricism and positivism. Some of the earliest and best-known work in this respect comes from Ann Oakley (1981, 1979) and Sandra Harding (1987, 1986). A useful overview of ideas and issues can be found in Letherby (2003).

was first 'discovered', current thinking about how it 'worked', what might cause it, the advantages and disadvantages of available treatments and what was (and wasn't) known within biomedicine. The summary I offered Wanda would have looked a little something like this:

> The word *endometriosis* comes from the Ancient Greek, meaning – literally – an abnormal condition of the uterus (Older 1984: 5). In biomedicine the disease is usually defined as a condition characterised by the presence of a substance similar to endometrial tissue – the tissue that lines a woman's uterus each month in preparation for the implantation of a fertilised embryo – in places outside the uterus (Phillips and Motta 2000: 3). At the conclusion of a woman's monthly menstrual cycle, if she has not fallen pregnant, the endometrial tissue lining the uterus will bleed and shed; this is a woman's period. In women who have endometriosis, the tissue situated outside the uterus does not shed, but still responds to the hormones that trigger bleeding and shedding. The tissue often bleeds and swells. Lesions, cysts, nodules and scar tissue may develop and cause severe cramping, bleeding and pain. Large masses called "adhesions" can also develop in such a way that organs that should not normally stick together become stuck and cause considerable pain. (Cooke and Trickey 2002: 6)

In many ways, I offered Wanda the kind of introductory *disease overview* that often appears in medical and self-help books about the disease, and that one might expect to find at the start of a book such as this one. My overview would, no doubt, have omitted some things (such as the longstanding claim in some sectors of biomedicine that endometriosis is a 'career women's disease'), but the basic 'facts' would have remained. In the case of endometriosis, those basic 'facts' would have included, at the least, that it was a disease specific to women, gynaecological in nature, connected to the menstrual cycle, relatively 'new' and on the rise, especially in the West. In addition, I would have explained that although endometriosis is of uncertain aetiology and incurable, a variety of treatments are available to women, each of which is designed to improve women's health, with varying degrees of effectiveness. In the years after that interview with Wanda, I became increasingly sceptical about even those most basic 'facts' about the disease, or at least, what it means to speak uncritically of 'facts' – for reasons that will become clearer as this book progresses.

Uncertainty, Mess, Complexity and Contest

Most obviously, perhaps, endometriosis is a disease exemplified by an unusually high degree of uncertainty, mess and contestation, so that even if it were *preferable* to produce a list of basic 'facts' about the disease, or a neat overview, it would not necessarily be *possible* to do so. There is, for example, uncertainty about some of the key features of the condition. This includes the fundamental assertion that endometriosis is a gynaecological condition peculiar to women. There is evidence of the disease being found in men, for instance, as well as remote locations including the lungs, knees and brain (Fukunaga 2012; Nezhat, King, Paka, et al. 2012; Agarwal and Subramaniam 2010; Giannarini, Scott, Moro, et al. 2006; Sarma, Iyengar, Marotta, et al. 2004; Beckmann, Pintado, Leonard, et al. 1985; Martin and Hauck 1985; Pinkert, Catlow and Straus 1979).[2]

Although endometriosis is still often characterised as a 'gynaecological' condition, there is a notable trend within endometriosis medicine to use more expansive terminology when describing the condition, so that the disease is now frequently described as – variously – an 'immune disorder', 'environmental disease', 'hormonal disorder', or 'genetic condition'. These classifications are not necessarily mutually exclusive, either, so that, it may be claimed, endometriosis is one or more of these 'things' at the same time.

In recent years there have also been attempts to revisit several longstanding assumptions about the disease's history, incidence and prevalence, with potentially widespread implications for how we understand endometriosis and its subjects. This has arguably led to even more instability and confusion. Debate rages about when the disease was first 'discovered' or recorded in the canon of medical literature, with most literature suggesting that the Bohemian physician von Rokitansky founded the disease in 1860, whilst elsewhere (Knapp 1999) it has been suggested that the disease was first documented in 1690 by Daniel Schroen (see, for a discussion, Batt 2011).[3] There are also debates about how long, prior to its 'discovery', women may have suffered from the disease. Nezhat, Nezhat and Nezhat (2012: 1) recently suggested that reports of women's 'hysteria', from antiquity to Freud, may in fact represent undiagnosed cases of endometriosis. In re-examining historical depictions of women's mental illness and wandering wombs, as well as witchcraft, lovesickness, nymphomania and more, the authors explained that:

> By applying [a] broader set of criteria we were able to uncover substantial, if not irrefutable, evidence that hysteria, the now discredited mystery disorder presumed for centuries to be psychological in origin, was most likely endometriosis in the majority of cases … If so, then this would constitute one of the most colossal mass misdiagnoses in human history, one that over the centuries has subjected women to murder, madhouses, and lives of unremitting physical, social, and psychological pain. The number of lives that may have been affected by such centuries-long misdiagnoses is staggering to consider, likely involving figures in the multiple millions.

---

2   I am indebted to Matthew Rosser for collating some of this literature in his endometriosis blog: http://endo-update.blogspot.com.au/2011/11/theres-something-you-dont-see-everyday.html, accessed 3rd May 2013.

3   In addition, Benagiano and Brosens (1991) claim that the condition was more likely discovered by Cullen.

The authors concluded that endometriosis 'appears to be an old disease that has affected women for millennia' (Nezhat, Nezhat and Nezhat 2012: 56).[4] What these few examples reveal, then, is that depending on which historical account one believes, endometriosis is either an ancient disease or a very new one.

By extension, another area of major disagreement involves the scale of the 'problem'. While some estimates suggest that less than 100 million women are affected worldwide, others put the estimate at double that. More recently, Nezhat, Nezhat and Nezhat (2012) suggested that somewhere between 900 million and 1.5 billion women are affected. Against this it has also been suggested that endometriosis might not even be a 'disease' at all (see Evers 2010).[5] In all of these ways, endometriosis is a disease that might be best described as ontologically uncertain, messy, complex and contested. These various 'features' of the disease (and the field of endometriosis medicine more broadly) raise a number of important questions. What, for instance, are the implications of this uncertainty and of competing claims about the disease? How does this uncertainty, mess and instability play out in endometriosis medicine? How does it factor in to medical practice? How do these many different ideas about the disease shape responses to it? How do women diagnosed with the condition engage with this complexity, mess, uncertainty and instability? Curiously, can we even speak about 'endometriosis' medicine/practice/etc. when there appears to be a lack of consensus about the central ontological referent? How does medicine handle this instability? Is some consensus being forged from amidst the chaos, confusion and debate? If so, what is the nature of such consensus, how is this achieved, and why might these various processes and practices (in securing a central ontological referent) matter? As these few examples and questions reveal, the need for a critical study of endometriosis seems almost self-evident. This book represents an initial attempt to come to grips with the significance of this uncertainty, instability, mess and contest, and with various other features of this symbolically potent and politically significant disease. I will argue that these overlapping phenomena – of uncertainty, mess, complexity and contest – are epistemologically, politically, and materially significant, with a range of implications for how the disease is managed and treated, and with consequences, of course, for women who live with the disease. But before I explore these ideas any further, I want to say something further about the many other reasons why more (and more critical) research into endometriosis is necessary.

---

4   Although there has been little historical research regarding the existence of endometriosis among women prior to the 'discovery' of the condition in 1860, evidence of its existence has been said to date as far back as 1600 BC (Henderson, Riley and Wood 1991).

5   I explore some of these ideas in Chapter 2.

Why Study Endometriosis?

A full-length social scientific study of endometriosis is, I suggest, both urgent and desperately overdue. In order to understand what has been done to date and why more work is needed, some historical context might first be useful. Initially, endometriosis was thought to be an extremely rare condition, with just 20 reported cases of the disease in the medical literature to 1920. Thinking about (and interest in) endometriosis has changed dramatically since that time, however, so that somewhere between 5 and 15 per cent of all women are now thought to suffer from it (Nezhat, Nezhat and Nezhat 2012; Overton, Davis, McMillan, et al. 2002; Weir 2001). Putting aside questions of contestation and uncertainty, if these figures are to be believed, endometriosis is even more common than both breast and ovarian cancer (Phillips and Motta 2000: 6). Endometriosis now runs second only to uterine fibroids as the most common reason that women undergo gynaecological surgery (Overton, Davis, McMillan, et al. 2002: 15). The most widely reported symptoms associated with the disease are menstrual pain (dysmenorrhoea),[6] pain during sexual intercourse (dyspareunia), pain during bladder (dysuria) and bowel movements, and heavy bleeding during the menstrual period and at other times of the month (menorrhagia) (Simeons, Hummelshoj and D'Hooghe 2007). Women may suffer from some or all of these symptoms, or from none. In many cases, endometriosis can result in infertility (Cox, Ski, Wood, et al. 2003a: 201), although the mechanism by which this occurs is uncertain (Dougherty 2004: 133; Sutton and Jones 2004: 6). An estimated 30–40 per cent of all women with endometriosis are found to be infertile (Phillips and Motta 2000: 15). In many cases the disease recurs after treatment, including hysterectomy. In other cases the disease disappears spontaneously and may or may not recur. No treatment has been found to completely eliminate recurrence (Gao, Outlety, Botteman, et al. 2006: 1562). It is for all of these reasons that endometriosis has been variously described as 'puzzling' (Ballweg 2003d: 1), an 'enigma' (Thomas 1993), 'mysterious' (Holloway 1994: 24), a 'conundrum' (Molgaard and Gresham 1985), 'complex' (Gao et al. 2006) and 'enigmas wrapped in riddles' (Jaffe 2004: xv).

The apparent surge in diagnoses in the latter half of the twentieth century, often noted anecdotally, has led a number of writers to describe endometriosis as a 'hidden' epidemic or an 'epidemic ignored' (Ballweg 2003b: 376; Vanderhaege 2000; Anthony 1996; Koski 1995; Holloway 1994). The world's first and most prominent self-help group for sufferers of endometriosis, the

---

6 In medicine, there are two different types of dysmenorrhoea. 'Primary dysmenorrhoea ... is menstrual pain without identifiable pathology; secondary dysmenorrhoea is painful menses with underlying pathology' (Callahan, Caughey and Heffner 2004: 293). Whether a woman is thought to be suffering from primary or secondary dysmenorrhoea is a matter of clinical interpretation. Endometriosis is classified as a clinical example of secondary dysmenorrhoea.

American Endometriosis Association, has called the disease 'a modern epidemic' that 'appears to be growing rapidly'.[7] Its apparent status as both a gynaecological disease and a 'modern epidemic' renders endometriosis as a distinctive condition, insofar as *it is perhaps the only global epidemic pertaining to women*.[8] In and of itself, this feature justifies the need for more work on the disease, but there are many other reasons why research into endometriosis is needed. In general terms, endometriosis has a rich and fascinating history, insofar as it has been characterised by a range of theories about what causes the condition and the kinds of women who may develop it (Missmer and Cramer 2003). Historically, for example, endometriosis was known as the 'career women's disease', based on an assumption that only career-oriented women who 'thought' too much were prone to develop it (Carpan 2003). A range of similarly problematic claims about the psychological attributes of the disease population have traditionally featured in the biomedical literature, although all too rarely have they been the subject of academic scrutiny. There is a long history, as well, of women's complaints of menstrual pain being dismissed and/or trivialised within biomedicine, so that many women with the disease have struggled to achieve the necessary credibility to have their complaints taken seriously. Importantly, as we shall see, endometriosis is also a thoroughly gendered and highly stigmatised condition, one that is negotiated around the meanings of blood, menstruation, pain, fertility and infertility, within a context, as I have already mentioned, of biomedical uncertainty, confusion, debate and instability.

The notion of endometriosis as a modern epidemic has gained traction over recent years, with the term being applied with increasing frequency in medical literature, self-help literature and the media. Despite this, however, public awareness of the condition remains relatively low. According to Last (1995, quoted in Green, Swartz, Mayshar, et al. 2002), an epidemic is:

> The occurrence in a community or region of cases of an illness, specified health
> behavior, or other health-related events clearly in excess of normal expectancy;
> the community or region, and the time period in which cases occur, are
> specified precisely.

This, of course, is just one definition. The notion of 'epidemic' is highly contested and contestable, as Green, Swartz, Mayshar, et al. (2002) explain in their article 'When is an Epidemic an Epidemic?' In that paper, the authors note that the word 'epidemic' comes from the Greek, where *epi* means upon and *demos* means

---

7   http://www.endometriosisassn.org/news.html

8   This description of the epidemic may appear to contradict my earlier concerns about how the disease is understood and defined, especially given evidence that endometriosis has been located among men. My point, however, is that such findings have been largely dismissed and/or understood as anomalies within biomedicine, having little or no impact on understandings of the disease as specific to women and/or gynaecological.

people. In this sense, the word 'epidemic' roughly described 'that which falls upon populations' (Last 1995 quoted in Green, Swartz, Mayshar, et al. 2002). So what – precisely – is understood to be 'falling upon' the population as a result of this burgeoning 'new' epidemic? Judging by the language used in endometriosis discourses, the term 'epidemic' tends to be deployed in a very specific set of ways. Typically, endometriosis is said to be at 'epidemic' proportions, with a sharp and historically recent increase in disease prevalence. Although claims have been made about the distribution of the epidemic across populations, it has been suggested that the disease burden is higher in Western nations (and increasingly so), and that the very 'nature' of the disease is changing, not just in terms of the severity and range of symptoms being experienced, but the shifting manifestations of the disease, with more women at younger ages being impacted, for instance. In one publication, produced by the American Endometriosis Association (2009), the incidence of endometriosis is said to be 'rising dramatically':

> Doctors have puzzled over why incidence of endometriosis, which was considered relatively rare even in the early 1980s, has been skyrocketing. Affecting at least 7.5 million women and girls in the United States and Canada, it afflicts millions more worldwide.

In the same publication, the authors dismiss possible, alternative explanations for the current epidemic:

> Advances in diagnosis and reporting do not explain the current epidemic rates of endometriosis. Greater awareness fails to explain documented increased rates of hysterectomies due to endometriosis, most notably in teenage girls.

These are bold – and disturbing – claims that raise a number of questions about contemporary medical care, disease awareness and practice. Beyond this, however, I suggest that questions also need to be asked about the implications of making assertions such as these – literally, metaphorically and materially. What does it mean to speak of a 'modern' epidemic that is peculiar to women? What does it mean to describe a disease as 'puzzling', or to speak of a 'skyrocketing' disease incidence? One of the central arguments that I will make in this book is that the making of claims about the status of a disease (which may include claims about its incidence and prevalence) is never an inert or neutral activity. Instead, articulations about disease are fundamentally and thoroughly implicated in the materiality of that disease, generating certain rewards, but also costs. These ideas are central to the book, and I will come back to them shortly.

One of the most common ways for assessing the 'significance' of a disease and/or the need for research is in assessments of the overall health burden of the condition. In a systematic review of research examining the economic burden of endometriosis, Gao, Outley, Botteman, et al. (2006) found a paucity of studies exploring the overall cost of the disease. Extant studies tended to address the costs associated with management of specific symptoms, or the cost of specific treatments, such as GnRH agonists (Gao, Outley, Botteman, et al.: 1569).[9] The authors concluded that 'the economic burden of endometriosis to society is substantial' (Gao, Outley, Botteman, et al. 2006: 1568). These findings were largely supported in a subsequent systematic review (Simeons, Hummelshoj and D'Hooghe 2007).[10] Assuming that endometriosis affects 10 per cent of women of reproductive age the authors estimated the annual costs of endometriosis in the USA in 2002 at approximately US$22 billion. This can be compared with the annual cost of diseases comparatively similar in terms of medication expense and medical/surgical options, such as Crohn's disease, with an estimated annual cost of $865 million and migraines, with an estimated annual cost of $13–17 billion. Cost estimates of diseases are important for public policy purposes because they can 'underline the importance of a disease to society when considered alongside its impact on morbidity and mortality and when compared with the economic burden of other diseases' (Simeons, Hummelshoj and D'Hooghe 2007: 396). Despite the apparently relatively large economic burden of endometriosis, public health policy interest in the disease remains extremely low. Unfortunately, this lack of interest is not confined to the public policy realm; there are surprisingly few academic studies exploring various aspects of the disease.

Previous Research into Endometriosis

This is not to say that the disease has been entirely neglected by scholars, however; indeed, there is an important body of existing work that explores several important questions, employing a range of methods (e.g. Denny and Mann 2007; Whelan 2007, 2003, 2000, 1997; Ballard, Lowton and Wright 2006; Emad 2006; Denny 2004a, Denny 2004b; Ballweg 2003a, 2003b, 2003c, 2003d, 2003e, 2003f; Cox, Ski, Wood, et al. 2003a; Cox, Henderson, Anderson, et al. 2003b; Cox, Henderson, Wood, et al. 2003c; Barnard 2001; Capek 2000; Shohat 1998).[11] In existing studies, the topic that has been given most attention is the period *before* women's diagnosis with endometriosis. There is a specific reason for this: women experience an average delay of nine to ten years between the onset of symptoms and diagnosis with the disease (Stratton 2006; Arruda, Petta, Abrao,

---

9   In a separate study, Simeons, Hummelshoj and D'Hooghe (2007: 401) concluded that studies examining the cost of endometriosis also suffered 'from a number of methodological limitations, thus producing biased costs estimates'.

10   See also, more recently, Simeons, Dunselman, Dirksen, et al. (2012), where the authors found that loss of productivity and decreased quality of life were two of the largest factors in the high economic burden of endometriosis.

11   I have also published on aspects of women's experiences and the disease (Seear 2009a, 2009b, 2009c, 2009d).

et al. 2003; Ballweg 2003a: 355; Husby, Haugen and Moen 2003). Several studies have therefore examined women's experiences of the diagnostic delay and the possible reasons for it. In the case of endometriosis, the biomedical standard is that the disease cannot be confirmed to be present in the uterus until it has been identified by a qualified physician (Brewer 1995: 51). Any diagnosis is merely 'suggested by the history', requiring the physician's imprimatur as it is 'corroborated by the pelvic examination and verified by culdoscopy, biopsy and laparoscopy' (Kistner 1971: 443). For women as patients, the patient's reported 'history' that may be suggestive of endometriosis is predominantly pain-related (Ballweg 2003a: 344; Phillips and Motta 2000: 12). In order to obtain a diagnosis, therefore, women's accounts of pain must first be accepted by medical professionals. It appears that this represents a stumbling block for many women for a range of reasons, one of which is the trivialisation of menstrual pain among some health professionals. Previous research has also generated important insights into the experience of being diagnosed with endometriosis, offering a sense of the overall experience of living with the condition. A number of these studies are limited, however, in important respects.

Some of these limitations were addressed in a systematic review of the research exploring women's experiences with endometriosis. In that review, Denny and Khan (2006) identified eight (published) qualitative studies exploring women's experiences. A number of themes common to the eight studies were identified, including a focus on the experience of pain, the impact of treatment, the delays in diagnosis and the impact of endometriosis on personal relationships and sexuality (Denny and Khan 2006: 505). However, of the eight qualitative studies examined, the authors found that only two moved beyond a simple description of the data (with quotations or examples) to an analysis and interpretation of the meaning and significance of that data (Denny and Khan 2006: 504). They also argued that with some exceptions, the studies could be 'characterised as not having an appropriate design, usually because questions posed were vague, or because the design was not made explicit' (Denny and Khan 2006: 505). With the exception of Emma Whelan's invaluable work (2007, 2003, 2000, 1997), emerging out of a doctoral dissertation on the disease, most studies have focussed on only one dataset, such as focus groups, and a narrow set of issues. Only a handful of studies have been conducted which give voice to women and most of these have been published only in recent years. As Elaine Denny (2004a: 646) rightly points out, therefore, 'the thoughts and feelings of women with endometriosis about their future lives do not feature in the previous literature'.[12] As well as this,

---

12   Some of the main findings from the literature are that women diagnosed with the condition can experience concern, worry, anxiety, self-blame, financial and relationship difficulties and a reduced quality of life (Manderson, Warren and Markovic 2008; Denny and Mann 2007; Strzempko Butt and Chesla 2007; Abbott, Hawe, Clayton, et al. 2003; Jones, Kennedy, Barnard, et al. 2001; Wright and Shafik 2001; Garry, Clayton and

most work to date has been largely atheoretical, failing to critically engage with several key assumptions and assertions that characterise the field. To the best of my knowledge, therefore, this book is the first full-length social science work on endometriosis produced anywhere in the world. It represents a modest attempt to encourage more critical thinking about several claims and practices pertaining to one of the world's most common – and burdensome – health problems for women. In the next sections, I outline the key questions this book seeks to address and my theoretical approach.

The Social Construction of Reality

The starting point for explaining the theoretical framework that I will use in this book is in the conventional approach to understanding health, illness, epidemics and disease, or what might be broadly termed as an objectivist and realist approach. As Arun Saldanha (2003: 420) explains:

> Realism ... ultimately believes that the physical and even social world itself discloses what it is, and can be fully explained if only scientists look hard enough.

In this sense, a realist approach to endometriosis would see the disease as a 'natural' phenomenon or biological 'fact' that exists prior to its 'discovery' by biomedical science. From this perspective, endometriosis exists outside of the scientific processes through which it is located, isolated, categorised and even named. So, even though endometriosis may have only been *discovered* in 1860, it was always already there, as a 'natural', essential, biological disease entity. Realism is therefore best understood as an approach that posits a world that exists 'out there', waiting to be unveiled by science and medicine. Crucially, realism holds that the 'real world' is ontologically stable, singular and coherent.

In contrast, social constructionists seek to challenge fundamental and taken-for-granted assumptions about the world, including assertions about the 'natural-ness' and inevitability of 'facts' (Hacking 1999). As regards medicine,

---

Hawe 2000; Bodner, Garratt, Ratcliffe, et al. 1997; Ballweg 1997; Ballweg 1992). It was found that fear, anger and depression are common features amongst sufferers. Women feel isolated and alienated through their experience, with some of these studies suggesting that sufferers can feel overwhelmed and powerless in the face of the disease. It was found that this is partly a consequence of delays in diagnosis of the condition and partly the result of treatment at the hands of the medical profession, where most women report that their general practitioners have not taken their symptoms seriously (Carlton 1996; Hadfield, Mardon, Barlow, et al. 1996). Women with endometriosis are also considerably incapacitated. In a United States National Health Interview Survey, for instance, it was found that half of the women who reported suffering from endometriosis were bedridden because of the disease for an average of 17.8 days during the 12 months before the survey (Kjerulff et al. 1996 cited in Weir 2001: 1201).

constructionists emphasise the social, cultural and political dimensions of science and medicine, in ways that effectively operate to denaturalise disease.[13] Deborah Lupton (2003: 12) explains social constructionism as:

> an approach which questions claims to the existence of essential truths. What is asserted to be "truth" should be considered the product of power relations, and as such is never neutral but always acting in the interests of someone. The social constructionist perspective argues, therefore, that all knowledges are inevitably the products of social relations, and are subject to change rather than fixed.

Social constructionism has been applied to a range of topics, issues, phenomena and 'things'. Ian Hacking (1986), for example, has explored the various ways in which 'people' are constructed, a notion that includes both the making of specific types of people (such as 'the pervert'), and the very notion of individual subjects as discrete social actors or entities. Importantly, the social constructionist approach can also be extended to ideas, ideologies, 'biology' and 'nature', so that even taken-for-granted claims about the natural body (e.g. that there are two sexes, and these two sexes exist as a product of nature) can be challenged (see Goode and Ben-Yehuda 1994). In one of the best-known examples of a social constructionist approach to science, Bruno Latour and Steve Woolgar (1979: 243) argue that:

> Scientific activity is not "about nature", it is a fierce fight to *construct* reality. The *laboratory* is the workplace and the set of productive forces, which makes construction possible. Every time a statement stabilizes, it is reintroduced into the laboratory (in the guise of a machine, inscription device, skill, routine, prejudice, deduction, programme, and so on), and it is used to increase the difference between statements. The cost of challenging the reified statements is impossibly high. Reality is secreted.

Once reality has been constructed, it tends to become 'taken for granted' and 'difficult to dislodge' (Hahn 1995: 70). As Nelly Oudshoorn (1994: 139) argues in her history of sex hormones, these difficulties emerge because the social and cultural dimensions of knowledge production and the construction of reality tend to be forgotten, submerged and disguised:

> One of the reasons why science succeeds in convincing us that it reveals the truth about nature is that the social contexts in which knowledge claims are transformed into scientific facts and artefacts are made invisible. Science makes us believe that its knowledge claims are not dependent on any social context. During the development of science and technology the established links with the worlds outside the laboratory are naturalized.

---

13   See also Berger and Luckmann (1966).

According to Sarah Nettleton (2006), social constructionism is now considered to form an important conceptual framework – if not *the* most important conceptual framework – in the sociology of health and illness. Its popularity may emerge from the belief that social constructionism is:

> wonderfully liberating. It reminds us, say, that motherhood and its meanings are not fixed and inevitable, the consequences of child-bearing and rearing. They are the product of historical events, social forces, and ideology. (Hacking 1999: 2)[14]

Because of these apparently fundamental differences in approach, realists and social constructionists are usually seen as being vastly at odds with one another. This war of ideas seems to be grounded in a set of seemingly insurmountable paradoxes, where:

> One person argues that scientific results, even in fundamental physics, are social constructs. An opponent, angered, protests that the results are usually discoveries about our world that hold independently of society. (Hacking 1999: 4)

The Science and Technologies Studies (STS) scholar Annemarie Mol has argued that in spite of claims to the contrary, social constructionism and realism are not actually as different as we might think. Crucially, both modes of thinking share a common flaw, with a tendency to portray objects as ontologically *singular* and *stable*. Within realism, objects (e.g. substances such as drugs, or diseases) are understood to be *stable*, insofar as they have *consistent* and *predictable* 'natural' properties and attributes that exist prior to their enrolment in social relations, as well as efforts to understand, discover or otherwise deal with them (Duff 2013; Dwyer and Moore 2013; Fraser and Moore 2011). Similarly, within social constructionism:

> The term "construction" was used to get across the view that objects have no fixed and given identities, but gradually come into being. During their unstable childhoods, their identities tend to be highly contested, volatile, open to transformation. But once they have grown up objects are taken to be stabilized. (2002: 42)

The implication here is that the materialisation of an object (or objects) through 'construction' happens as a once-off, never-to-be-repeated process. And so here lies our immediate problem: constructionist frameworks simply will not do in the study of endometriosis. In other words, as I have already noted, endometriosis

---

14   Although, of course, this claim depends on both how liberation is defined, and on whose perspective one is taking. Social constructionism may be liberating in some instances and for some mothers, but not for those fathers who have traditionally benefited from discourses pertaining to maternity, childbirth and childrearing arrangements.

knowledge and practice remains 'under construction',[15] in a state of uncertainty and flux, characterised by continuing uncertainty, contest and instability (including a debate about whether it is even a 'disease' to begin with). Endometriosis does not have a 'fixed' or 'given' identity (even if such a thing were possible, and even if claims are often made to the contrary). Importantly, this is not a problem exclusive to endometriosis. Annemarie Mol's point is that the central assumption of constructionism (that objects are ontologically fixed, singular and stable) is fundamentally unsustainable. And so it is on these questions – around the 'nature', 'making' and stabilisation of reality – that Mol's approach differs from that of constructionists.[16] Drawing from insights generated in her own ethnographic work on anaemia (1999) and later, atherosclerosis, Mol argues that although objects *are* made, 'maintaining the identity of objects requires a *continuing* effort', and that over time the ontology of objects might 'change' (2002: 43; my emphasis). In this respect, the 'construction' of reality is better understood as a dynamic and ongoing process, where objects are constituted through continuing, iterative practices, rather than a set of processes that take place over a finite period and eventually come to a halt.[17] In this sense, Mol's approach is also a 'performative' one, following the feminist and queer theorist Judith Butler (1993, 1990). What

---

15 In this respect I am borrowing a phrase used by Jaclyn Duffin (2005: 83) to describe hepatitis C. In my work with Suzanne Fraser on hepatitis C (Fraser and Seear 2011), we also used this term to describe the uncertainty and flux pertaining to that disease. It seemed fitting to use it again here.

16 To be clear, this is not the only (or indeed the main) criticism levelled at social constructionists. Constructionists are often accused of overplaying the role of language and discourse in the production of reality and underestimating (or even ignoring) the role of matter (see Barad 2007, 2003, 1998). The importance of matter will be explored later in this book. As well, one of the other main limitations of social constructionism is in its tendency to reify 'the social'. What I mean by this is that social constructionism often assumes that there actually *is* something relatively stable and coherent called 'the social' and – crucially – that 'the social' pre-exists the process of 'construction'. Bruno Latour wants us to approach the notion of the social as a 'specific domain of reality' (2005: 4) much more critically, especially when it is mobilised as a way of explaining various phenomena, or as a means of asserting a unidirectional causal relationship (i.e. that a given problem is *caused or constructed by or within 'society'*). Addressing the broader question of what sociology is and what it can do (as opposed to narrower questions about social constructionism), Latour calls for a new approach: one in which we focus instead on 'the tracing of associations', where the 'social does not designate a thing among other things … but *a type of connection* between things that are not themselves social' (2005: 5). To put it more simply, Latour urges us not to *begin* with the social, but to *end* with it. Not only, then, does Latour's criticism challenge some of the key components of 'social' constructionism, it opens up new opportunities for thinking through cause and effect. It also raises the possibility, as we shall see, that objects are *made* in some way that exceeds the social, but also – crucially – that the social 'itself' is made through connections – or 'traces' made by new associations. Tracing the making of objects allows us, in Latour's terminology, to 'reassemble the social'.

17 See also Fraser and Seear (2011).

I mean by this is that reality – or, in Mol's terms, *realities* – are *made* through repetitive actions, gestures, movements and articulations (a theoretical approach that Butler refers to as 'performativity'). Crucially, Mol also argues that objects are fragile, with a 'complex present', and that the ontology of objects 'may differ between sites' (2002: 43). Using the example of anaemia, Mol argues that:

> The reality of anaemia takes various forms. These are not perspectives seen by different people ... neither are they alternative, bygone constructions of which only one has emerged from the past ... they are different versions, different performances, different realities that co-exist in the present. (1999: 79)

So, for example, different discursive practices may materialise different versions of anaemia (or atherosclerosis), or perhaps even endometriosis. Moving away from the language of constructionism, Mol argues for an approach to ontology as 'multiple', 'enacted' and changeable, as opposed to singular, constructed and stable. These observations are significant for a number of reasons. Most importantly, in emphasising objects as inherently changing and changeable, and the making of objects as an ongoing process, Mol opens up a set of interlinked possibilities:

- that diseases differ as between sites and in space/time, with different implications;
- that the ontology of disease is constant iteration, meaning that any number of actions, gestures, movements, practices and articulations are suddenly materially, politically and ethically significant;
- that just as realities are made and sustained through continuing efforts, reality is changeable and thus might be made anew;
- that by attending to specific practices, articulations, gestures, and more, we might simultaneously intervene in the making and maintenance of ontologies, so that new versions of disease may materialise.

This brings us to the deeply political function – or the 'ontics', as she prefers – of Mol's approach. This requires me to say something about the relationship between the making of disease and the making of subjects.

Subjects, Objects and Politics

These implications arise out of the idea, explored within social constructionism, feminism, post-structuralism and queer theory (e.g. Butler 1993, 1990), that subjecthood and subjectivity is also *made*, rather than natural, fixed, or given in the order of things. In other words, subjects, like diseases, do not possess stable, inherent 'attributes' that precede human action or social relations, but are made and remade within them. As well as this, the making of objects and of subjects is closely connected and mutually co-constituting, so that 'within contemporary neo-liberal societies the making of disease is also necessarily the making of subjects, of rights and responsibilities' (Fraser and Seear 2011: 1). This is perhaps best illustrated by some examples from the critical literature on HIV/ AIDS, which Dennis Altman (1992) has called 'the most political of diseases'. The advent of the HIV/AIDS epidemic offers perhaps the starkest example of the fundamental links between politics, the materiality of disease, subjects, rights and responsibilities. As we now know, the HIV/AIDS epidemic is not exclusive to any one sector of the population, although it was initially thought to be an exclusively 'gay disease' or 'gay plague' (see Treichler 1999, Waldby 1996). Initial public health responses to the epidemic were limited by this idea, but also by a set of deeply politicised assumptions about sexuality, sexual practice, the body, gender and risk. So, for instance, while the epidemic was originally assumed to be exclusive to gay men, a set of hypotheses – and later, assumptions – about the causal links between gay sexual identity and 'practice' were thought to be implicated in how the disease was 'caused' or spread. These might include, for example, gay men's apparent propensity towards unprotected sex and the fundamentally 'promiscuous lifestyles' of gay men.[18] Ideas about the disease cohort fundamentally shaped public health responses to the epidemic in the early years, with gay men emerging as the target of public health campaigns. Guided by these hypotheses, normative evaluations, assumptions and stereotypes, public health campaigns were dominated by a desire to contain the very contaminability of gay men's bodies and to control seemingly problematic behaviours amongst the gay male populus. So, gay men were suddenly responsibilised, enjoined to engage in 'safe sex', curb their promiscuous 'tendencies', refrain from a range of sexual activities and more. As the virus spread, the assertion that gay men were implicated in the nascent epidemic also took hold in both the public and biomedical imaginary, a phenomenon that undoubtedly further stigmatised an already highly stigmatised and marginalised population. In this way, gay men were 'effectively treated by much public health discourse *as if they themselves were the virus*, the origins of infection' (Waldby 1996: 13), to devastating effect.[19] The key point here is that the HIV/AIDS epidemic proceeded on the basis of an assumption that its principal 'subjects' (gay men) possessed certain (foundational) attributes and qualities that preceded medical knowledge and practice, as well as numerous other discursive practices and formations. Crucially, these assumptions and claims were materially productive, insofar as the 'promiscuous' and 'contaminated' gay male

---

18   There were also, of course, many more assumptions about the way that the gay male body might be implicated in the manifestation and materiality of the epidemic, several of which are discussed by Waldby (1996) in her excellent book *AIDS and the Body Politic*.

19   According to Catherine Waldby (1996), the initial emphasis on gay men as the origin of infection and target of public health intervention eventually gave way, as understandings about the disease shifted. Importantly, however, heterosexual men continued to be overlooked in public health campaigns, with heterosexual women being subjected to demands to help control the spread of the virus.

subject emerged as an 'effect' of the epidemic. In other words, as Michel Foucault (2002: 54) reminds us, discursive representations and practices 'systematically form the objects of which they speak'.

There can be no doubt that these initial assumptions about sex, gender and sexuality also shaped public health outcomes and the very materiality of the epidemic, a materiality which might ordinarily be understood, according to the orthodox realist model, as developing 'naturally'. What I mean by this is that opportunities to control and even minimise the rate of new infections in the initial stages of the HIV/AIDS epidemic were almost certainly lost, by virtue of assumptions about what the disease was, how it was spread, who was spreading it, what we could expect (by way of preventative action) from at-risk and affected populations and how else it might be managed. These early assumptions therefore had – and continue to have – major global implications for both heterosexual and homosexual populations, in that the pattern and scale of the epidemic would likely have been different had things been done otherwise. Most obviously, the failure to effectively engage with heterosexual communities was a major oversight, especially because, as we now know, HIV/AIDS was never exclusive to the gay population. There have also been major implications for people living with AIDS, including, in particular, those gay men who were subjected to a set of inaccurate assumptions and unrealistic expectations (regarding both transmission and prevention) in the initial years. In this respect, HIV/AIDS offers an unfortunate – and unfortunately bleak – example of the mutually constitutive relationship between discourse, disease/epidemic, the subject and 'the social', insofar as ideas about each have worked to shape the other. In this book I want to suggest that similar processes are at work in relation to endometriosis. I want to highlight the co-constitutive dimensions of material-discursive relations, the stigmatising and marginalising dimensions of these processes, and, using critical theory of the kind just described, consider how and where we might intervene in the disease in order to produce new, less stigmatising versions of endometriosis and the endometriotic subject. The question, then, is *how* we might go about exploring this. These questions pertain to modes of thinking, writing and researching in academic work, the relationships between discourse and realities, and the format of this book.

Research and Writing (Or, Performance and Politics)

John Law is a well-known STS scholar and regular collaborator with Annemarie Mol. In his books *Aircraft Stories* (2002) and *After Method* (2004), Law makes a number of important observations about writing and researching that have implications for how I want to approach the present analysis. Speaking first about method, Law (2004) suggests that the STS emphasis on enactment and multiplicity demands a new approach to research (see also Law and Mol 2002). According to Law, conventional social science methods have long been predicated upon realist assumptions of the kind I described earlier: the belief, that is, that there is a world 'out there' for social scientists to capture. Research methods tend to be understood as the means through which that reality will be 'captured'. Although a comprehensive review of Law's ideas is beyond the scope of this book, the tradition of observational research within the social sciences (including especially, sociology and anthropology) offers a useful way of highlighting the main threads of his critique.[20] Marshall and Rossman (1989: 79) define observation as the 'systematic description of events, behaviors, and artifacts in the social setting chosen for study'. This seemingly simple definition of method obscures a set of crucial assumptions. These include the notion that the world exists independently of the researcher who merely 'describes' it, and – following Mol (2002) – that the object/s of analysis are stable, coherent and singular.[21] Law's point is that traditional research methods do not tend to be sensitive to reality as multiple and enacted, nor, crucially, to the 'mess, confusion and relative disorder' (2004: 2) of the world. Arguably, social science methods actively suppress that complexity and mess, whether through the establishment of research questions, the selection of objects, the use of certain methods, the processes of coding or the handling of data (dismissing or downplaying, for example, so-called anomalies). This, again, is an especially pertinent observation with regards endometriosis (because it is not a very 'neat' disease).[22] As a disease thoroughly imbibed with uncertainty, instability, mess and contestation, it is crucial that researchers adopt theoretical frameworks and methods that attend to these complexities, rather than simply ignoring, dismissing, or trouncing all over them. Worse still, it is crucial that researchers not be tempted to 'resolve' or 'fix' the mess; instead, we should look carefully at how that mess is handled, rationalised, smoothed away or otherwise dealt with, as this is likely to reveal much about the various objects and subjects under investigation. Although Law is less clear on what research might look like 'after method', it seems clear that attending to complexity, chaos and mess are crucial, as, perhaps, are approaches that combine methods and data-sets across space and time. In *Organising Modernity* (1994), Law offers another suggestion, encouraging researchers to move from the study of 'nouns' to 'verbs', and from 'things' to 'processes' (because 'things', of course, are merely the 'effects' of iterative processes).

---

20   For a more detailed discussion of Law's work on method, and a discussion of how it might be taken up in research on a particular field (alcohol and drug use), see Duff (2012).

21   Similar observations have been made before, of course – a point that Law (2004) himself acknowledges. Within the field of sociology, for example, there is a considerable body of work on 'reflexivity', including analyses on the way that a researcher's self/body/subjectivity/emotions and more shape the research encounter, process and findings (see, for example, Ellingson 2006; Adkins 2002; Finlay 2002, 1998; Reger 2001).

22   Of course this is not a phenomenon specific to endometriosis. Law's point is that 'neatness' and 'order' are themselves enactments.

These ideas surface again in *Aircraft Stories* (2002), where Law dedicates considerable time to questions around 'doing' and 'process', with a focus on the ethics, politics and 'effects' of different forms of writing. For Law, there are two possibilities regarding 'how texts relate to the world'. The first is 'that they tell about and thus represent a version of reality' (2002: 6). This approach rests upon a fundamental distinction between the text itself and what it represents. He explains:

> If we think of writing in this way, then we distinguish between texts on the one hand, and what they represent on the other. The latter become something separate, out there, prior, removed. This means that we may stand outside and describe the world, and that when we do so we do not get our hands dirty. We are not in the world. (2002: 6)

The second way of understanding how texts relate to the world is more reflexive: 'that telling stories about the world also helps to *perform* that world' (2002: 6). Extending this observation to the subject of his book, the TSR2 aircraft, Law explains that the effect of his approach to texts is that 'no matter how stories are told about this aircraft … they do not simply describe something that happened once upon a time. They are, rather, also a way of helping to perform the aircraft. The stories *participate* in the aircraft'. Law is making two slightly different but interrelated points here. Like Mol, he is suggesting that reality does not exist prior to 'representations' about it. By extension, reality is neither stable nor fixed. Texts, to use Annemarie Mol's language, enact reality – they *make* things, as opposed to simply *portraying* them. This involves a departure from the traditional (and decidedly more modernist) notion of the author, which posits them as the knowing subject, documenting objective reality. In this respect, Law's approach to texts is based upon a rejection of at least three ideas: the first is in distinctions between the knowing subject and the observed object, the second is that a stable reality exists that can be separated from the perspectives of the authors that create texts and those who read them, and the third is that only certain forms of writing are political. Indeed, all forms of writing are always already political.

Following John Law (2002), then, one of the central ideas in this book is that all forms of writing – indeed, all forms of textual representation and articulation – do not simply *represent* the subjects and objects with which they deal, but participate in the *materialisation* of them. Writing performs the world. This applies to all forms of writing, including academic writing. So just as the stories that Law tells about the aircraft that is the subject of his book work to enact that aircraft, so do the stories that I choose to tell in this book operate to enact endometriosis. Importantly, Law's observations pertain to both form and content. On the question of form, Law (2002: 55) argues that stories about technologies, science and medicine often adopt a storytelling style that 'starts at the beginning and moves to the end', a form of storytelling that he calls *plain history*. Taking as his case study the development and decline of the TSR2 aircraft project, Law goes on to suggest that:

there is obviously no such thing as "plain history". All history, "plain" or otherwise, is a narration and a performance. It makes, distributes, and links things together, bringing them into being and asserting their significance (or otherwise) by chaining them into possibly chronological sequences. (2002: 55)

The connections and links that are made in writing constitute a 'kind of truth regime', with a range of 'consequences'. In this sense, both the form and content of writing are fundamental to the making of reality. This is an important idea for at least two reasons. First, it implies the need for critical analyses of the written form (which includes, in the present context, key sites of articulation for endometriosis such as medical literature and self-help books). Secondly, however, it raises questions about how we might approach our task as analysts, insofar as academic writing has a central role to play in the production of the world.

How Should We Write about Endometriosis?

In writing about diseases, especially diseases that are as uncertain, contested, complex and messy as endometriosis, it is tempting to try and produce a neat account of things for the reader, assuming, as I do, that both the large volume of literature about the disease and its complex history will be mostly unfamiliar. In my earlier work exploring the history of endometriosis, I always grappled with the question of how to achieve this, assuming, of course, that it is the job of an author to produce a 'neat' account of that type. What is the best way to condense the vast scientific and medical literature published over many years? How can I explain the range of theories about the disease? Should all theories about endometriosis be discussed, or only those typically considered as the main (or most plausible) ones? How can I reproduce this information in a form that will do justice to the complexity of the disease's history as well as the connections between past, present and future, as I have come to understand them? How to deal with inconsistencies in logic of the kind I mentioned at the outset of this chapter (e.g. that although generally considered a 'gynaecological' disease, endometriosis sometimes 'mysteriously' appears elsewhere in the body)? What choices should be made in the presentation of women's stories? Given the complexity of the disease and the range of issues experienced by many women (including pain, infertility, diagnostic delays, experiences of treatment, and more) how are decisions to be made about what to include, and what to leave out? How might these choices shape understandings of the disease and its subjects? These are just some of the questions that need to be asked.

A common approach within medical sociology and medical history is to produce a *chronological* account of disease, so that readers might follow how ideas about a condition have 'changed, 'evolved', or 'progressed' over time. There are certainly many advantages to producing a chronological account of that nature. It should, for one, enable readers to follow the flow of ideas over time; to see how earlier (prior) disease concepts have informed later ones, in sometimes subtle, sometimes more obvious ways. Alternatively, one might produce a *thematic* account of a disease: carefully locating within the myriad of details about the disease a series of connections, links, trends and patterns in thinking, themes which might themselves be linked in sometimes subtle, sometimes more obvious ways. Unfortunately, many conventional medical and scientific histories of disease adopt either or both techniques. I say 'unfortunately' here, because both styles of writing have the potential to function as a kind of 'plain history', or as an *overview*, a notion that has been problematised within STS.

Mol and Law (2002) have written together on the significance of the 'overview' as a style of writing. They argue that although simple overviews (like the one I offered Wanda) may seem innocuous, they actually involve a set of important choices that work to constitute reality. Overviews typically omit certain things, presenting a version of reality as self-contained and neat. In this way, overviews dispel chaos and create an 'illusion' of order. Through the choices we make in the production of overviews, we often erase complexities. So, for example, any overview that describes endometriosis as a chronic gynaecological condition produces order and (the illusion of) coherence at the expense of complexity, contestation and uncertainty (by avoiding reference, for example, to those cases where the disease has been found in other 'parts' of the body, or in men). Overviews therefore operate to deny both the complexity and multiplicity inherent to reality. Importantly, accounts of this kind are part of the process by which reality is enacted and stabilised. More often than not, one thing that chronologies do is produce an ordered account of science as 'progress', by documenting clinical 'insights' and research 'breakthroughs', examining ways in which old ideas gave way to new ones, and examining the role of technological innovations in knowledge progression. Although not all chronologies follow this exact approach, elements of this appear in many of them. Where a chronology either purports or functions to 'track' developments in the interplay of science, technology and knowledge over time, it will almost always work to produce those developments as a form of 'progress'. In this sense, disease analyses that utilise a chronological approach very often operate to valorise medicine and science, producing and reproducing them as rational and heroic enterprises. One of the ways they do this is by producing space and time, for space and time, as I will argue, are effects of the historico-medical chronology. Or more precisely: chronologies are one of the means by which space and time are produced and reproduced. The way we write medical histories (which may include the way we set out and order disease theories), may create an 'illusion' of order in the history of a disease, and in so doing, produce medicine and science *as order*. The same can be said for thematic histories, although such histories will usually achieve the same ends by a different means. For these reasons, I have decided to avoid both the thematic and chronological approaches to disease in this book.

The Pinboard-Pastiche Method

If chronological and thematic approaches metaphorically and materially produce medicine and science as rational enterprises, and if we take seriously the notion that medicine and science are not always or inherently such, what form might a more critical account of disease take? First, in keeping with the overall approach of the book and the intellectual and philosophical commitment to avoiding totalising accounts of the disease and its subjects, this book does not purport to comprise a comprehensive review or overview of the history of endometriosis, nor of the evolution of scientific ideas about the disease and its subjects. Among other things, I do not consider all of the extant theories about endometriosis and/ or practices in relation to it. I also do not consider all aspects of women's lived experiences with the disease, nor all of the practices that work to materialise the disease/epidemic.[23] Instead, my book involves a necessarily selective approach to the disease, in which I explore key figures, articulations and practices in relation to it, as well as aspects of how women living with the condition experience it. The choices that I have made about what to include and exclude are not intended to be a reflection on the significance or otherwise of particular aspects of the disease, although I recognise, following Law (2002), that these choices will inevitably perform a version of endometriosis. The particular version of endometriosis that is performed in this book will be further shaped, I suggest, by any claims I make about the relationships between ideas, theories and data.

In recognition of this complexity, John Law (2002, 2007) poses a new way of approaching both research and the narrative, based upon the metaphor of the pinboard. So, as Law (2007: 134) explains:

> The rationale for pinboards is that somewhat but not entirely random stuff gets stuck on them ... These bits and pieces, all juxtaposed ... are partially connected. Physically they lie on a surface, there are lots of them, and they overlap too. (There isn't much space on the pinboard. Things are jostling together.) But (this is important) they are partially *disconnected* as well.

The pinboard is a 'pastiche' (2002: 189), Law argues, where objects lie alongside one another, without any 'obvious hierarchy or narrative' (2007: 135). He goes on to say that the paradox of the pinboard is that:

> A two-dimensional but otherwise unstructured surface is potentially quite permissive about the character of relations between the pieces arrayed upon it. Its two dimensions produce not two dimensions but many. (2007: 135)

23　There are a plethora of sites where these issues could be examined. These include media coverage of endometriosis, social media, creative art therapy and autobiographical writing on the illness. A fascinating example of the latter is *Giving up the Ghost* (2003): the memoir of acclaimed British writer Hilary Mantel.

Importantly, the construction of the pinboard involves a number of conscious choices about form and content, much like a book. These include what to incorporate and what to omit, as well as how to order items. Placing something at the heart of the pinboard, for example, may perform that object as more 'central' and significant to the phenomenon in question than any other item on the board. It may also imply a set of relations between that item and all of the others. Pinboards can perform realities – but they have the potential to constitute them differently, especially through careful attention to these details (think how a pastiche-style approach may differ in both 'look' and effect to a conventional chronological account of disease, for instance). Importantly, a pinboard is 'not a view from nowhere' (2007: 135), but a way of challenging, making and re-making the world. In this sense, following Law (2007), I understand the main features of a pinboard-pastiche to be one in which:

1. Phenomena are performed as non-hierarchical, where everything is more or less equivalent;
2. Metaphysical claims to singularity are dismissed in favour of a reality enacted as multiple;
3. There is no claim that the pinboard is a 'complete' account of the phenomenon in question;
4. There is non-coherence. Tensions are allowed to co-exist, instead of being smoothed away. In so doing, the pinboard again performs and acknowledges ontological complexity; and
5. The overlaps between the objects on the pinboard are understood as affecting one another in potentially important ways, but the nature and significance of these connections remains open-ended, open to interpretation and – crucially – open to change.

The Focus of this Book

This book is a critical study of endometriosis using the experimental qualitative methodology of pinboard-pastiche. It traces various processes pertaining to the disease and the epidemic, with an emphasis on how the disease is articulated, lived, negotiated, materialised and performed, and how, in turn, these arrangements – as a set of material-discursive practices – are significant. In what follows, I assemble an account of the various complexities and political dimensions of the disease as a phenomenon. Drawing upon insights from STS and feminist theory, in particular, the book explores the following questions:

1. What is the significance of the idea that endometriosis is a 'modern epidemic'?
2. How and in what ways do concepts of 'agency', 'gender', 'matter', 'nature' and 'culture' figure in accounts of endometriosis?

3. How is the endometriotic 'subject' enacted in biomedical and self-help discourse? How might ideas about the subject operate to shape the disease and/or epidemic?
4. In what ways might the deployment of these concepts work to constitute the materiality of endometriosis, both as 'disease' and as 'epidemic'?
5. What is the significance of the considerable uncertainty, instability, mess and debate surrounding endometriosis (for medical knowledge and practice, the materiality of the epidemic, and women diagnosed with the condition)? How, in other words, are these material and discursive 'features' of the disease productive?
6. What insights can be drawn from this study to inform policy and practice pertaining to the disease?

These questions are explored across three datasets: medical journal articles charting the history and identification of endometriosis, self-help books written for women with the condition and in-depth interviews with women who have been diagnosed with the disease.[24] I also consider ancillary material that appears in research and advocacy materials, especially in the first chapter.

The first chapter of the book examines how endometriosis is enacted in medical research and advocacy. It is among disease activists that some of the most sensational claims about endometriosis have been made. These include the notion that endometriosis is both on the rise and a 'modern epidemic', and becoming more severe. I examine the symbolic and material dimensions of these claims. Looking at two particular instances from medical activism, I argue that endometriosis figures as a literal and symbolic 'crisis of the modern', and that the declaration of the endometriosis epidemic performs a set of intersecting, symbolic, material and ethical concerns surrounding the gendered, natural, human, traditional body. Endometriosis emerges as material and symbolic threat to tradition, nature and the 'human', in ways that are highly gendered and thoroughly political. Most of all, the discursive framing of endometriosis among some activists simultaneously reflects and reproduces the importance of ordered modernity, although, as I argue in that chapter, understandings of both order and the 'modern' change over time.

The second chapter moves into new territory, with an analysis of endometriosis in the biomedical literature. One of the persistent features of the biomedical literature is the production and deployment of theories about endometriosis, which includes theories about the mechanisms of the disease, as well as the main 'traits' and 'attributes' of the disease cohort. In this chapter I examine the significance, in particular, of the plethora of theories that surround the disease, arguing that the simple practice of theorising plays an important role in constituting subjects and social relations. I focus on the way that disease theories produce and reproduce a

---

24 The original study was approved by the Monash University Human Research Ethics Committee. All of the names and other identifying details of participants in the study have been changed.

set of ideas about gender, nature, culture and agency, arguing that medical theories perform medicine as ultimately heroic and progressive, despite medicine's inability to come to grips with key facets of the disease/epidemic. In this sense, Chapter 2 also articulates one of the key concerns of this book: that uncertainty, incoherence, tension, inconsistency and debate have productive dimensions and are centrally implicated in the making of the world.

The third chapter engages with the form and content of the endometriosis self-help literature. In keeping with the book's overall commitment to exploring 'multiplicity', this chapter considers how an entirely unique genre of writing (one that differs in key respects from biomedical writing) enacts its own version/s of endometriosis. Focusing on a selection of texts available to women with the disease, I consider how self-help books frame both the disease and its subjects, and how agency and subjectivity are performed and distributed therein. I argue that self-help literature performs endometriosis as inherently mysterious and complex, at the same time as it enacts it as singular, coherent and stable. These tensions and paradoxes co-exist in the self-help literature, alongside a highly problematic version of agency whereby women are constructed as both responsible for and capable of managing their illness. I consider how these versions of ontology and agency complicate women's experiences of the disease, introducing, for the first time, interview data from women living with the condition. I conclude with a set of recommendations for revising the approach to disease and agency in self-help books.

In the fourth and fifth chapters I turn my attention to interview material collected from in-depth interviews with 20 women who have been diagnosed with endometriosis. The fourth chapter focuses on women's experiences of treatment, while the fifth chapter examines a range of issues pertaining to women's experiences of living with the disease, including how the notion of 'self-care' figures in their lives. The decision to order the chapters in this way is a deliberate one. In the biomedical imaginary, treatment is often understood as the end point of the illness trajectory. In the case of endometriosis, however, women's engagement with treatment does not always end in triumph; indeed, treatment often complicates women's experiences of illness. The fourth chapter explores some of these factors, and the relationship between treatment and subjecthood. I argue that treatment intra-actively constitutes a range of subject positions, including, crucially, the kinds of subjects that medicine purports to be treating. This analysis is especially significant in the case of endometriosis because the 'traits' and 'attributes' of endometriotic subjects are usually understood to pre-date their enrolment in medicine, and to play a significant causal role in the development of the disease. This analysis therefore raises questions about causation and the medical encounter, with potential implications for how we view the epidemic. The fifth chapter extends some of these observations even further through a consideration of how an ethic of self-care emerges and plays out in women's lives. I argue that women with endometriosis find themselves at the juncture of an almost impossible paradox: enjoined to care for themselves and manage their illness as a form of putative liberation, many discursive practices associated with self-care operate to produce women as weak, irrational, sick and responsible for their own predicament. I consider some of the challenges women face in negotiating these tensions, and conclude with a call for a more critical approach to self-care. The book concludes with a set of reflections on the disease, and some questions that I hope will be taken up in future work.

Chapter 1

Crisis of the Modern:
On Advocacy, Research and the
Rise of Endometriosis

Declarations of epidemic are declarations of war.

(Waldby 1996: 1)

Despite its apparent status as the one truly global epidemic to impact women, there has been surprisingly little critical investigation of the dual notions, used so often in relation to the disease, that endometriosis is both an 'epidemic' and a '*modern* epidemic'. Each of these assertions seems to demand detailed analysis. To my knowledge there has been no critical exploration of the deployment of these terms, how and where they are used, what they might mean and – perhaps more importantly – how they function once deployed. Epidemics, of course, have already been the subject of much academic attention. There is, for instance, a well-established and sophisticated body of work pertaining to the HIV/AIDS epidemic (e.g. Sontag 2001; Treichler 1999; Altman 1986). In one of the seminal works in that field, *AIDS and the Body Politic*, author Cathy Waldby describes 'Declarations of epidemic [as] declarations of war' (1996: 1). In biomedicine, she suggests, epidemics are 'crisis points in the Darwinian evolutionary struggle' between the human and nonhuman. They are typically declared, according to Waldby, when 'too many bodies succumb' to colonisation by a viral or bacterial population (1996: 1). Epidemics, therefore, are a symbol of fear and panic, an ontological threat, insofar as the epidemic places, in the biomedical imaginary, at least, the very existence and status of the 'human' at risk (Waldby 1996: 1). Waldby's work suggests that questions about boundaries and binaries (such as human/nonhuman) are necessary and intrinsic to any critical study of epidemics. But how are these questions relevant in relation to endometriosis? What added meaning do these questions take on – or how might the questions we ask and the answers that we generate – be shaped by the fact that endometriosis is not simply an *epidemic*, but so, it seems, a specifically *modern* one?

It is here – with the question of what it means to speak of, write about, practise and treat a modern epidemic – that I want to begin my analysis in this book. Although I agree with Waldby's argument that declarations of epidemics are declarations of war, I want to suggest that the nature of the 'war' will likely differ depending on the specific epidemic in question. For instance, the kind of war articulated via the HIV/AIDS epidemic, saturated as it is with the politics of gender, sexuality and race, among other things, will differ from the kind of war declared via the endometriosis epidemic. If nothing else, the endometriosis epidemic is specific to women's bodies, so a different set of issues and anxieties are likely to be involved. This chapter explores these differences and similarities, with a view to isolating the specific and localised dimensions of the battles that are being materialised via the endometriosis epidemic. This includes, in particular, how each of the various components of the war (nature, culture, human, nonhuman) are enacted. In this sense, I am particularly concerned with how discourses about the endometriosis epidemic work to enact specific versions of (and ideas about) the battle between nature and culture, human and nonhuman, and the wider symbolic and material significance of those enactments. In what follows, I also consider the significance of the specifically 'modern' characteristics of this war and what this means for the wider analysis that I will undertake in the remainder of the book.

These issues are explored through accounts about the disease from the field of medical advocacy and research. I have chosen to look at these issues via medical research and advocacy because it is here that declarations of the endometriosis epidemic first appeared and are most often repeated. My focus in this chapter is with the way that two particular accounts of the epidemic – taken from the field of medical research and advocacy – perform the disease and the epidemic. What do these accounts take the epidemic to mean? What are the causes of the epidemic? And why should we be concerned about it? Is a war being declared? If so, who is at war? The two accounts I have chosen to examine appear between 30 and 50 years apart. This is a very deliberate choice on my part, because I am interested in how claims about the rising epidemic diverge and overlap, and any continuity and flux in the ideas contained therein. These accounts, I will argue, are connected in several important ways. Among other things, both involve what are generally understood to be important figures in the history of the disease: advocates who have done much to help bring attention to the increasing incidence of the disease, and to explore the possible reasons for that trend. Each account renders the 'causes' of the epidemic differently, but in ways that are interrelated. Importantly, as we shall see, the 'modern' figures in both instances as central to the spread of the disease, although the 'modern' is performed differently. The two accounts that I explore in this chapter are also connected through their relationship with binary logic. Binary logic, broadly speaking, is a form of rationality involving the use of dualisms or opposing pairs (such as order/chaos, or good/evil). Binary logic underpins Western thought and practice, with significant political, ethical and material implications. In what follows, I argue that accounts of endometriosis perform several binary pairs and that the various 'limbs' of each pair are enacted as being at war with one another. This, I will argue, is both symbolically potent and materially significant. Finally, I explore one of the other main ways that both accounts are connected – through their reference to and engagement with monkeys. Monkeys feature prominently in each of the accounts I will examine here, and yet their place in medical research/advocacy and the emergent 'epidemic' has been hitherto overlooked. I explore how both of these accounts handle and utilise the monkey, and how the monkey's appearance in each works to produce the disease, the epidemic and the war. In this sense, my deliberations on the role of monkeys demonstrate the importance of attending carefully to the various figures that feature in medical research and advocacy – including those that are often marginalised – with a view to exploring their role in the production of knowledge and the material world. In focusing explicitly on the role of the monkey in this way, I explore alternative ways of understanding the function of medical research and advocacy in relation to disease and epidemics, arguing that it is fundamentally implicated in the making of both.

In this chapter I will argue that medical research and advocacy perform endometriosis as what I will call '*a crisis of the modern*'. Put simply, the declaration of the endometriosis epidemic is a declaration of multiple, intersecting, symbolic, material and ethical concerns surrounding the 'gendered, natural, human, traditional' body. Endometriosis emerges as a literal and metaphorical point at which various 'threats' to the gendered, natural, human, traditional body are enacted. Through the disease, the dangers thought to be posed by culture, the nonhuman, modernity and industrialisation surface and coalesce. Although some of these dangers simultaneously enact gender (and thus emerge as *gendered hazards*), a few of the dangers that I will discuss here have no specific relationship to gender. Using my two accounts from medical research and advocacy as exemplars of this process, I also argue that the form of the 'modern' – and thus, the nature of the 'crisis' – changes over time. I consider the importance of this continuity and flux. As a disease hitherto neglected among most social scientists, endometriosis emerges as a condition deserved of serious academic attention, not least because of its symbolic and material status as 'crisis'. It is, indeed, an always already gendered, highly politicised and ethically charged phenomenon. In what follows, I introduce a range of theoretical concepts that are relevant to the analysis in this chapter, before I move on to explore accounts of the disease/epidemic.

Binaries and Boundaries

Endometriosis is a disease thoroughly shaped by and through boundaries – by the notion, that is, that all things have their right and proper place, by notions about separation, containment, limitations and frontiers. As well as being underpinned by ideas about 'bodies' as bounded and regulated, endometriosis materialises boundaries and concerns about the inappropriate transcendence of them. Take, for example, the following three definitions of the disease found in medical literature. These definitions are typical of those that appear in other literature where definitions of the disease are offered. In each of these examples, notions of 'inside', 'outside' and the inappropriate transcendence of boundaries are conspicuous:

- Endometriosis is tissue that somewhat resembles the *inner* lining of the uterus, but that is located *outside of the uterus where it doesn't belong* (Redwine 2009: 6; my emphasis).
- Endometriosis, defined by the *ectopic presence* of endometrial glandular and stromal cells *outside the uterine cavity*, is a benign yet common gynecological disorder affecting from 1 to 22 per cent of women of reproductive age (Guo 2004: 157; my emphasis).
- Endometriosis is defined as the implantation of endometrium-like glandular and stromal cells *outside their normal location* in the uterus (Varma, Rollason, Gupta, et al. 2004: 293; my emphasis).

In each of these examples, endometriosis is defined through a certain kind of 'binary logic' – an idea often associated with the French philosopher Jacques Derrida. Derrida (2002, 1976) argued that Western logic is dominated by and derived from a series of binary oppositions (or pairings). Examples of binary pairs include: mind/body, human/non-human, reason/emotion, objective/ subjective, object/subject, nature/culture, authentic/inauthentic, passive/active, order/chaos and – as with the three examples that I have included here – inside/ outside. In binary logic, the meaning of each term in a pair derives in part from its relationship to the other. As well, terms in a binary are positioned as mutually exclusive and hierarchical, so that one term enjoys a privileged and dominant status, while the other is always already deprived and subordinate. So, as Elizabeth Grosz (1989: 27) explains:

> Within this structure the opposed terms are not equally valued: one term occupies the structurally dominant position and takes on the power of defining its opposite or other. The dominant and subordinated terms are simply positive and negative versions of each other, the dominant term defining its other by negation.

To take an example: 'Body is ... what is not mind, what is distinct from and other than the privileged term' (Grosz 1994: 3). As well as the relational and mutually exclusive functions that we can identify as *within* each pair, there is an important relational function *between* binary pairs. Binary pairs, put simply, are 'relationally aligned' (Grosz 1994: 4). In this sense, the 'mind' is not simply the dominant term in the mind/body dualism, but symbolically linked to other dominant pairs, including reason, culture, authenticity and order. At the same time, the 'body' is symbolically and literally devalued – first through its association with the more valued figure of the 'mind', and then through its symbolic association with its relationally aligned binaries, such as emotion, nature, inauthenticity and chaos. Crucially, as Elizabeth Grosz (1994) has pointed out, the mind/body opposition has also been historically correlated with the male/female binary. In this way, men are symbolically associated with the mind, activity, objectivity, culture, authenticity, order and reason (among other things), while women are symbolically associated with the body, passivity, subjectivity, nature, inauthenticity, chaos and emotion.

To the extent that each of the latter is produced as subordinate, women are always already symbolically and literally devalued. In this regard, binary logic has a political and ethical function.

To bring these ideas briefly back to endometriosis, I want to suggest that the disease can already begin to be understood as a thoroughly politicised and debased object. This is because, to begin with, the very definition of the disease is forged through binary logic, involving as it does the idea that tissue spreads 'outside' a set of established, normative boundaries. In this regard, tissue that goes 'where it doesn't belong' (Redwine 2009: 6) – as the very hallmark of the disease – is a signifier of absolute subordination and abjection, and of the disease's greater symbolic significance as a state of thorough disavowal. This is obviously hugely significant, and a matter to which I will return.

Binary logic has received much academic attention in recent decades, in fields as diverse as semiotics, critical theory, feminism, race and cultural studies, critical nursing and queer theory. As well as focusing on the *existence* of binary logic, some of this work has sought to destabilise assumptions about the foundational status of binaries. In much conventional Western thought and practice, for example, the separation between 'nature' and 'culture' is taken as obvious or given. According to this line of thought and practice, men enter into the world as fundamentally and essentially different from women. The existence of distinctions such as these is already patently obvious, as is the way in which the categories are defined and organised. In addition, the body is understood as self-evidently natural, while the clothing that adorns it is understood as always already cultural. As an extension of this, the status, for example, of 'nature', is understood as predominantly stable: there is no sense in which components of 'nature' or the 'body' can move between binary categories; skin is always 'natural' and part of the 'body', while a pair of trousers is not capable of being re-categorised as part of the 'body', or as 'natural' rather than 'cultural'. There are several reasons why we need to critically engage with assumptions such as these, however. First, and perhaps most obviously, the uncritical acceptance of the prior status of these categories and the boundaries between them tells us nothing about how these very same classes and boundaries are *formed*. By what means is the body defined as distinct from the clothing that adorns it? How is the body assigned to the category of nature when all manner of other 'things' (earrings, reading glasses, iPods, mobile phones) are not? These are important questions, of course, because of the potential for binaries to function politically and ethically.

Because, as I have already noted, binary logic operates ethically and politically (through, for instance, enacting some practices and/or subjects as devalued, while valorising others), the question of boundary *maintenance* is also crucial:

> Binary opposites, once established, do not remain uncontested. They exist in a constant state of flux as boundaries shift to include or exclude, repairing their fractures and eliminating instability. (Magdalinski 2009: 43)

To what extent do binary-boundaries change and/or remain constant? How does contest happen? How might we account for the disruption and/or maintenance of such boundaries? It is critical that we explore the question of how boundaries, assuming them to be mobile and fluid, are *formed, maintained* and *challenged.* Questions around the function, formation, maintenance and disruption of boundaries, as we shall see, are crucial to understanding both the formation of the endometriosis epidemic and the politics of the disease. Up until now, I have said little about the question of agency as it relates to binary logic, or to the question of how binary logic might be understood to *function.* This is an extremely important question, especially for the analysis that I undertake in the rest of the chapter, and it is a question to which I will now turn.

The Power in/of Binaries

It is not possible to speak about binary logic without addressing the interrelated concepts of agency and power. I have already implicitly touched upon these links, albeit briefly, through the seminal work of Elizabeth Grosz. As Grosz (1994) reminds us, binaries always function ethically and politically, through registering some 'subjects' as passive, chaotic and so forth, while others are rendered as active, ordered and rational. The point that Grosz is making here is that binaries are *productive*: they work to surface particular kinds of subjects and objects, states of being, characteristics and qualities. In this regard, binary articulations, insofar as they may bear politically and ethically, are a form of power. The meaning of each term in a binary pair, crucially, is forged through relation to its 'opposite'. Accordingly, our understanding of chaos is generated through reference to what it is not (order), and vice versa. Every manifestation of order, however it appears, helps reiterate and shape the meaning of chaos, while simultaneously securing its own meaning and form. Because the meaning and value of binary opposites are formed via a relationship of assumed and projected mutual exclusivity, the terms can never be said to pre-exist. Instead, they surface through a range of processes, including processes of iteration and reiteration. Judith Butler (1990: 37) argues that the processes by which these distinctions are formed tend to be 'effectively concealed' from view, so that they appear to be fixed and self-evident, even though they are discursive productions. Paying close attention, therefore, to how processes work to forge these distinctions is a crucial component of understanding how power is both effected and distributed.

Questions around binary logic, power and agency have been the subject of much analysis in the field of science and technology studies (STS), including, specifically, those STS scholars most closely associated with Actor Network Theory (ANT) (Latour 1987; Law 1987; Callon 1986). ANT is a complex and diverse body of work in which questions regarding binaries, agency and power have been explored in even more radical ways. I want to concentrate on just a few of the most salient aspects of ANT here, especially work that seeks to challenge and dissolve dualisms like those I have discussed so far. In particular, I am interested in the central idea, articulated by John Law (1999: 3), that:

> Entities take their form and acquire their attributes as a result of their relations with other entities. In this scheme of things entities have no inherent qualities: essentialist divisions are thrown out on the bonfire of the dualisms ... there *are* no divisions. It is rather that such divisions or distinctions are understood as *effects or outcomes*. They are not given in the order of things.

In ANT, this logic is applied 'ruthlessly to all materials – and not simply to those that are linguistic' (Law 1999: 4), so that, notoriously, neither 'humans' nor 'nonhumans' are assumed to be fundamentally distinct or different from one another, nor to possess any prior qualities. One of the main issues that ANT theorists have engaged with in this respect involves the question of agency, including who or what has the capacity to act upon the world. As Callon and Law (1997: 168) explain:

> Often in practice we bracket off non-human materials, assuming they have a status which differs from that of a human. So materials become resources or constraints; they are said to be passive; to be active only when they are mobilized by flesh and blood actors. But if the social is really materially heterogeneous then this asymmetry doesn't work very well. Yes, there are differences between conversations, texts, techniques and bodies. Of course. But why should we start out by assuming that some of these have no active role to play in social dynamics?

This thoroughly unique approach to the constitution of actors (or 'actants', as they are known in ANT) is a form of 'radical indeterminacy' in which nothing at all is taken-for granted: 'the actor's size, its psychological make-up, and the motivations behind its actions – none of these are predetermined' (Callon 1999: 181–2). In ANT, then, an 'object' that would otherwise be considered inert, nonhuman and passive – such as a door-stopper – is just as likely to be reappraised as active and skilful (Latour 1988a). The point, according to Latour, is not only that the boundaries between things categorised as 'human' and 'nonhuman' (and their relational alignments) are nebulous, but that they are, in many instances, unsustainable, not just ethically and politically, but practically. Abandoning pre-ordained distinctions, prescriptions and inscriptions of this sort enable a more comprehensive analysis of the social world (Latour 1988b) in which 'technologies', 'animals' and other 'nonhuman' objects are understood 'as valid and often consequential participants in technoscience and, by implication, other activities' (Caspar 1994: 845). As well, the ruthless and radical indeterminacy of ANT allows us, among other things, to attend to how binary logic emerges, is sustained, and disrupted.

Work that explores the constitution of the human/nonhuman binary and the question of nonhuman agency, respectively, is not without problems (e.g. Collins and Yearley 1992). One issue, for instance, involves the question of 'situated knowledges' (Haraway 1991) and the performative function of academic writing. Let's take Latour's work on the door-stopper (1988a) as an example. Here, Latour sets out to demonstrate the nebulous nature of the boundaries between categories such as 'human' and 'nonhuman' and the assumptions we regularly hold about the capacities of each. Latour approaches these issues by examining the competence and function of an everyday object – the 'door-stopper'. His starting point is that the door-stopper does not possess any inherent or assumed attributes or traits. Through observation, Latour looks at what the door-stopper *does*, concluding that it functions in ways that seem similar to that of a 'human' figure, like a doorman or doorwoman. In holding doors open, door-stoppers create a hole in a wall through which people can move, for example. Door-stoppers therefore operate in such a way that most of the time, people moving through the hole in the wall are able to freely pass without incident. Like a doorman/woman, the door-stopper emerges as agentive, competent and functional. It *does something*.

Although this example renders several important insights into the tenuous nature of assumptions about objects and their functions, Latour's analysis is not immune from criticism. Even as he strives to demonstrate that the door-stopper is neither inert nor incompetent, the division between human and nonhuman, subject and object never seems to be completely avoided; indeed, to some extent, it is reproduced.[1] This occurs in part because, as author of the paper, Latour seems to be actively bestowing agency and competency upon the door-stopper, thus reproducing the dichotomy of the knowing subject/object of knowledge that he sets out to challenge. These are no minor quibbles. Questions about who 'has' agency, who or what is an agent and who 'grants' agency to whom are matters of major concern. As we know, the configuration of subjectivity and/or the bestowal of agency upon some subjects and not others has historically functioned with catastrophic results, particularly for women, people who use drugs, and others, including Jewish, homosexual, 'gypsy' and disabled subjects of Nazi regimes. There may also be circumstances in which the attribution of agency – to both 'humans' and 'nonhumans' – operates with concerning effects, depending on how the 'agent' is configured and relationally situated. One potent example of this comes from the work of Monica Casper, whose particular interest is the status of the foetus in experimental foetal surgery. In such surgery, she argues, medical professions often understand foetuses to be subjects in their own right. Here, Casper argues that 'constructions of active fetal agency may render pregnant women invisible as human actors and reduce them to technomaternal environments for fetal patients' (1994: 844). There are also possible limitations to the extent to which agency should be attributed to nonhumans – in the case, for example, of pets such as cats. Despite the fact that cats may exercise agency at times, they might also be vulnerable and dependent as pets – they can be hurt by humans, kept indoors and starved to death (Casper 1994). Casper's point is that the extension of agency

---

1   Although for a discussion of some of these concerns, especially as articulated by Collins and Yearley (1992), see Callon and Latour (1992).

to nonhumans may sometimes be ethically problematic, especially if it functions to render nonhumans (like animals) as agentive, responsible and accountable in circumstances where such responsibilisation hardly seems appropriate.

Although Casper raises a series of important issues around the attribution of agency to (humans and) nonhumans, her analysis ultimately leaves open several questions. In wanting to attribute agency to humans but not to cats or foetuses, for example, Casper seems to ignore the fact that there might be circumstances where these 'nonhumans' should be afforded agency (Barad 2007). Although Casper argues that the attribution of agency is an inherently political process (with which I wholeheartedly agree), there is a sense in which she still wants to pick and choose how agency is distributed, thereby politicising the process of attribution in ways that mirror Latour's work. In my view, this does little to help advance things, or to transcend the problems that often manifest alongside binary logic. A way forward comes through the work of Karen Barad (2007: 216–17) who suggests that:

> The critical issue lies not in the attribution of agency to the fetus in and of itself, but in the framing of the referent of the attribution (and ultimately in the framing of agency as a localizable attribution) ... The construction of the fetus as a self-contained, free-floating object under the watchful eye of scientific and medical surveillance is tied to its construction as a subject under the law and the myth of objectivism ... the fetus is not a preexisting object of investigation with inherent properties.

Barad argues for an approach to the foetus as *phenomenon*, where the focus of analysis is upon how the idea that the foetus is a subject in its own right (as distinct from the mother) emerges to begin with. After this, she suggests, the focus should be upon agency, which includes the way that agency is constituted in and distributed via discourses and practices (since the meanings of agency are not stable or prior, either). This approach, like much work in ANT, works from the position that everything is radically indeterminate, including 'subjectivity' and 'agency' itself. It is with this approach in mind that I now turn to my two accounts of endometriosis from medical research and advocacy. In what follows, drawing upon the work of Grosz, Butler, Latour, Casper and Barad, I consider how medical research and advocacy produces subjects, objects and agency through articulations of the epidemic. I consider how the materialisation of each of these, following Butler, can be implicated in the production of a binary logic regarding the disease. Finally, I consider how the binary logic that surfaces via research and advocacy is connected – symbolically and materially – to notions of 'war', and what this means for our understanding of the disease more broadly.

Disobeying Nature's Rules

In the 1930s, American physician Joe Vincent Meigs was beginning work on endometriosis, which had only recently been formally named within biomedicine.[2] Now considered an important and influential figure in the history of endometriosis medicine (see Way 1964), Meigs eventually became a prolific writer about this 'new' disease throughout the 1930s and the next two decades. He appears in many historical accounts of the disease as a leading 'advocate' and crucial figure (Batt 2011). Following in the footsteps of another such figure in the history of endometriosis medicine, John Sampson, Meigs was interested in a range of issues, including what endometriosis was and why it developed in women, but also why, by his reckoning, endometriosis appeared to be on the rise. In a series of influential papers published during the 1930s, '40s and '50s, Meigs grappled with these questions and more. His earliest work appeared in an editorial in *Surgery, Obstetrics and Gynecology* (Meigs 1938). In a 1941 paper, Meigs provided a succinct summary of his central ideas about the disease, arguing that the condition was due:

> to the economic times we live in, and my plea is that patients with apparent infertility, evidences of underdevelopment, and older girls about to be married, be taught how to become pregnant and not how to avoid pregnancy, even though their finances are limited. The monkey mates as soon as she becomes of age, and has offspring until she can no longer have any or until she dies. Menstruation in this animal must be rare. As women have the same physiology it must be wrong to put off child-bearing until 14 to 20 years of menstrual life have passed. (Meigs 1941: 869)

Later that same decade, Meigs revisited these ideas:

> In nature certainly early child-bearing and frequent child-bearing is the usual thing. This may be prevented by some untoward circumstances, such as caging and domestication. Certainly some monkeys who menstruate, as women do, mate early following the menarche and have offspring, nurse, and then become pregnant again. In their natural habitat, they probably follow this sequence until they either physiologically can have no more offspring or die. This is what nature expects of animals. The human being does not carry out nature's rules. Our grandmothers and great grandmothers probably more nearly approximated the ways of nature than the modern women, at least up to World War II. (Meigs 1948: 798)

---

2   In a 1925 paper (Sampson 1925b) entitled *Heterotopic or misplaced Endometrial Tissue*, John Albertson Sampson first coined the term 'endometriosis'.

In his 1941 paper, Meigs shared his clinical observations about the demographic distribution of his patients. He had come to the conclusion that endometriosis was less common amongst 'less well-to-do patients' than private patients of a higher status (Meigs 1941: 872), a theme he asserted persistently and which was the subject of his most significant papers (Meigs 1941, 1948, 1950, 1953). One of his main concerns was that the 'less well-to-do' might eventually out-produce those of a higher social status. He lamented that women of the upper classes appeared to have 'a difference in attitude towards childbearing' (1948: 796) and urged doctors to offer special counsel to those women, urging them to reproduce. In a subsequent paper, Meigs (1953: 52) offered the following recommendation to doctors:

> It is also true that the men and women in the more successful, higher income group, excluding the hospital doctors, are the ones who reproduce themselves fewer times than do the less successful and the less well-educated ... It would seem from this that we must encourage our own families and our more successful patients and their families to marry earlier, and when they are married, to have children.

Meigs' call to encourage reproduction was targeted directly at the upper classes: note the way that he implored doctors to encourage reproduction amongst 'our own families' and 'our more successful patients' rather than those 'less successful' or 'less well-educated' who also suffered from the condition. It seemed that Meigs was not only – or perhaps, necessarily – speaking to doctors in their professional capacity when he urged them to share his insights about the relationship between 'delayed' childbearing and infertility. Instead, he was concerned to maintain the lineage of his 'own' class:

> There is a great need in these times for financial aid to *our* daughters and sons ... Help when they are young is very important and by supporting their marriages and helping the young wife have her family we will accomplish much more for the world than we will by trying to save for them when they get older ... They should be encouraged to keep our country populated by having children when they are young ... I hope that it may strike a responsive note among the members of the association. (Meigs 1948: 805; emphasis in original)

The emphasis upon marriage and childbearing amongst the successful classes was later reiterated when Meigs explained to physicians: 'I have advocated early marriage and early childbearing among *our people*' (Meigs 1950: 719; emphasis mine). Meigs took the firm view, therefore, that endometriosis was a disease specific to white, well-educated patients (see also, for example, Scott and TeLinde 1950). These are detailed and complex passages regarding the disease, and there is much to be said about them. I want to briefly defer my analysis of Meigs' work, and turn to a second – much more recent – account of the disease. I want to then consider alternative possibilities for reading these accounts of endometriosis and what they achieve.

Serendipitous Findings

The second account of interest is also a story about what endometriosis *is*, and involves a new set of claims about the disease as epidemic. This account begins in the 1980s. A Canadian physician named James Campbell, funded by the Environmental Protection Agency, had published a study detailing a possible link between endometriosis and polychlorinated biphenyls (or PCBs) in food (Campbell et al. 1985). Dioxins and PCBs are part of a class of components of substances called 'xeno-oestrogens'. Xeno-oestrogen is a component of a substance found in the environment, food, air and that mimics the hormone oestrogen in the body water (De Vito et al. 1995 cited in Rier, Turner, Martin, et al. 2001b: 147; Vanden Heuvel, Clark, et al. 1994). Humans are exposed daily to these substances (Rier, Turner, Martin, et al. 2001b: 147). The main way humans are exposed to dioxin-like substances includes diet (Zeyneloglu, Arici and Olive 1997: 309–10). The study reportedly generated little interest at the time (Whelan 2000: 414). Some years after the study was published, Mary Lou Ballweg, the co-founder and President of the American Endometriosis Association (a support group for women with the disease), made contact with Campbell and discovered that his was not the only study of this kind to have detected a link between endometriosis and toxins (Whelan 2000: 414). Ballweg discovered that a separate study had been carried out on a population of rhesus monkeys. As part of that study, the monkeys were exposed to high concentrations of a chemical called dioxin. In what has since been described as a 'serendipitous finding' (Guo 2004: 157), two of the monkeys died, and upon examination were found to have developed severe endometriosis (Whelan 2000: 414).

Ballweg contacted those involved in the second study, only to discover that their funding had been exhausted. The researchers were in the process of selling the group of rhesus monkeys that had been exposed to dioxin for the purposes of the study. Concerned that an opportunity to conduct further research upon the monkeys might be lost, Ballweg called an emergency meeting of the Endometriosis Association. The Association resolved to provide urgent funding to enable the researchers to continue their work, and sought donations so that the colony could be saved and the research extended (Whelan 2000: 414–15). The results of the extended study were later published in what became a widely cited study (Rier, Martin, Bowman, et al. 1993).[3] As well as opening up a new area of interest,

---

3   The Rier study is widely cited in both medical and lay literature as the seminal study establishing a relationship between endometriosis and toxins (e.g. Colborn, Dumanoski and Myers 1997: 181). A slightly earlier German study (Gerhard and Runnenbaum 1992) had also concluded that there was a relationship between endometriosis and PCBs.

the study was said to have 'quickly sent a shock wave through the endometriosis research community' (Guo 2004: 157). The Rier study is understood as having:

> galvanized many investigators to look suspiciously at dioxin, and spurred more animal studies on the link between dioxin exposure and endometriosis. It also prompted many genetic studies in search for deficiency in genes responsible for dioxin detoxification, which may predispose women to endometriosis. (Guo 2004: 158)

The basic premise of the study was that dioxins and PCBs affect the body's immune system in ways that restrict a woman's capacity to fight off wayward endometrial tissue (Rier, Martin, Bowman, et al. 1993: 437).[4] The exact mechanism by which exposure to such chemicals might cause endometriosis was not clear, however (Rier and Foster 2002: 161). Sutton and Jones (2004: 2) describe this recently developed theory as the 'endometriosis disease theory' or EDT, which posits that:

> genetic changes occur in predisposed individuals exposed to environmental risk factors such as dioxins and biphenyl pollutants. (Sutton and Jones 2004: 2–3)

This is not to say that endometriosis is a genetic disease (in the heritable sense, although that possibility has also been mooted) but rather, that exposure to dioxin and dioxin-like chemicals may disrupt endocrine and immune responses in humans (see De Vito et al. 1995 cited in Rier, Turner, Martin, et al. 2001b: 147). The relationship between chemicals and pollutants in the environment and endometriosis is not certain and to date there have been no studies 'definitively linking' chemicals to an increased risk of endometriosis (Giudice and Kao 2004; see also Guo 2004).[5] In this sense, the apparently 'serendipitous' findings by Rier and her colleagues remain controversial.

Alongside the emergence of the dioxin hypothesis, the notion that endometriosis was now a disease of epic and epidemic proportions has gained traction. These two developments are by no means coincidental. Indeed, the apparent rise in incidence of the disease has been interpreted by many health advocates as further evidence of the likely accuracy of the environmental

---

4 For more recent studies suggestive of a relationship between chemicals and endometriosis, see Buck Louis, Weiner, Whitcomb, et al. (2005); Rier, Coe, Lemieux, et al. (2001a); Rier et al.(2001b); Mayani, Barel, Soback, et al. (1997). The subjects of most studies exploring the possible relationship between chemicals and endometriosis are rodents although a small number of studies involve human participants and report evidence of a positive association (see Buck Louis, Weiner, Whitcomb, et al. 2005: 279).

5 This is because research carried out to date has generated conflicting results (Zeyneloglu, Arici and Olive 1997: 324). At least two studies have found no statistically significant association between exposure to dioxin-like chemicals and endometriosis (Pauwels, Schepens, D'Hooghe, et al. 2001; Lebel, Dodin, Ayotte, et al. 1998).

hypothesis. As the environmental hypothesis has been developed, it has reinforced the suggestion that endometriosis is on the rise and becoming more severe, probably through the increasing prevalence of environmental toxins in our everyday lives. Women's health advocates have taken up these issues, including, in particular, members of various endometriosis support groups, claiming that environmental toxins are centrally implicated in the developing epidemic. This process of mutual co-constitution is typified by the following statement from Mary Lou Ballweg (1995 cited in Whelan 2000: 416) who asks:

> Is it possible, based on the PCB study, to speculate that the disease of endometriosis might have been a mild, mostly tolerable disease in the past (except presumably for a few unlucky souls) that has become severe and distinctly intolerable with the additional effects of pollutants in our bodies? Perhaps these studies will help explain why there seems to be an epidemic of endometriosis worldwide in this century.

I now turn to a consideration of these two accounts of endometriosis.

Towards a Non-realist Approach

These descriptions of endometriosis – what I will call the Meigs and Ballweg accounts, for ease of reference – have been interpreted as significant for several reasons. First, as I have already explained, both of the key figures involved in these examples were at the forefront of efforts – albeit several decades apart – to raise awareness of the disease as a modern and growing epidemic. Excerpts from the work of Meigs – like those I have quoted above – are often referred to as evidence of his determined attitude and dedication to women's health. His work – while not uncontroversial – is also generally understood as playing a central role in raising awareness of the disease during the 1940s and '50s, and of bringing attention to the burgeoning epidemic. Papers like the ones I have quoted from here are thus primarily read as support for the historic importance of Meigs to the field as a whole, as well as being prophetic early accounts of the impending epidemic. Accounts of Ballweg's rescue of the rhesus monkey colony and the Rier publication to emerge out of it – including subsequent commentaries on this research – are understood in much the same way. Take, for example, the work of Stella Capek (2000), one of the only social scientists to look at the dioxin hypothesis. She argues that the emergence of the dioxin theory is a positive development which has led to a:

> reframing of endometriosis, one that locates causality not in the individual body of a woman, but rather in the "social body" ... This reframing questions not only past scientific "facts", but reallocates moral blame. Instead of pointing to bad

personal choices made by the selfish career woman, it links a woman's body to "a new species of trouble" (Erikson 1991) stemming from a toxic environment. (2000: 351)

She goes on to say that the environmental focus:

Provides an additional connection between women across national boundaries and the global approach itself has yielded important results that are reshaping knowledge about the disease, the frame through which it is interpreted, and, no less importantly, the experience of having it. (Capek 2000: 354–5)

Curiously, Capek's glowing endorsement of the dioxin hypothesis and her assertions about its 'effects' – including its effects on women with the disease – come without her having conducted any interviews with women with endometriosis. This is just one example of the way that the findings by Rier and her colleagues have been subsequently reported. It is also one of many accounts to suggest that the American Endometriosis Association has played a leading role in unearthing key scientific facts about the epidemic and the disease. Capek's account contrasts 'past scientific "facts"' with the more rigorous and reliable account of endometriosis that has now emerged. Here, the quotation marks purport to discredit several earlier, apparently less scientific theories about the disease. In this regard, the interpretations of the Meigs and Ballweg accounts by academics, journalists, self-help authors and others are largely consistent with a realist understanding of the world, a concept that I explored in the introductory chapter.

It has long been a curiosity to me that the Meigs and Ballweg accounts are interpreted as simply *reporting* upon the nascent epidemic rather than, say, *participating in the production of it*. Such interpretations are only feasible if we apply to both accounts a pre-existing set of assumptions about the subjects and objects that are involved, including assumptions about the meaning and distribution of agency and subjectivity. The point I want to make here is similar to the one made by Karen Barad in her discussion of Casper's work on experimental foetal surgery. To reiterate, Casper's research shows that the physicians who carry out such surgery understand foetuses to have agency, by virtue of their initial construction of the foetus as a free-floating object and subject in its own right. The attribution of subjecthood to the foetus is, in a sense, the enabling platform for all else that follows, including the way that agency is constituted and assigned, and the 'effects' of these designations. In a similar sense, accounts from medical research and advocacy often take for granted the prior status of the objects and subjects that circulate through them. These may include assumptions about any or all of the following:

1. Objects – what objects are being rendered visible through advocacy and research?
2. Subjectivity – who are the subjects involved in bringing the disease/ epidemic to our attention?
3. Agency – who is agentive in this work, and what is agency?

In what follows, I want to argue for a different approach to both accounts – one that assumes nothing about the 'subjects' and 'objects' contained therein, nor the meaning or distribution of agency. As with Latour's doorstopper, I approach these stories as a 'naïve' reader (Law 2002), without preconceptions about any of the figures in these accounts, including 'monkeys' and 'humans'. In the next sections, I examine the way these accounts enact several key binaries. I also look at the way each account performs 'agency' and assigns it to subjects and objects. Through a consideration of an alternative approach to these stories – *one in which monkeys are actors too* – I argue that the accounts operate to perform endometriosis and the endometriosis epidemic as a crisis of the modern. This is achieved, first, through the enactment of several binaries pertaining to the disease, most notably: human and nonhuman; nature and culture; modernity and tradition; and chaos and order. Insofar as binaries tend to be 'relationally aligned', as Grosz (1994: 4) reminds us, these binaries emerge as both connected and functional in important ways.

1. Humans, Nonhumans, Nature and Culture

As I have already explained, the content and significance of both accounts are frequently read in realist terms, with both Meigs and Ballweg understood as functional subjects whose work has helped to uncover 'facts' about the disease, including changes in the pattern of incidence and prevalence. There is, however, one grossly marginalised figure (subject? object?) that features in both examples – the 'monkey'. Curiously, even though monkeys figure centrally in both accounts, they have been afforded only marginal status in subsequent accounts of the disease, research and advocacy. In spite of the fact that Meigs juxtaposes monkeys with women in ways that arguably equate the two, there can be no doubt that Meigs' account also works to forge a distinction between them, primarily through the way in which his account performs agency and then assigns it to monkeys and humans in dissimilar ways. This is most clearly achieved in the passage, introduced earlier, in which Meigs claims that early and frequent childbearing is the 'usual thing' amongst monkeys. The only instance where this might not happen is where monkeys are '*prevented* by some untoward circumstances, such as caging and domestication' (1948: 798; my emphasis). Here, the suggestion is that procreation is predestined and inevitable amongst monkeys but for the imposition of external obstacles beyond the monkey's control. When Meigs speaks of this occurring within the monkey's natural habitat, he produces monkeys as animals that procreate with predictable regularity, where reproduction is both 'normal' and 'natural'.

The full significance of this becomes clearer when later in the same passage Meigs examines reproduction among human beings. In deliberating on 'monkeys' and 'humans' separately like this, Meigs immediately performs them as separate and distinct. This is the first thing that these accounts do, then. Like monkeys, women are obliged to 'carry out nature's rules' – nature 'expects' as much – and like monkeys, women may neglect to reproduce. Whereas monkeys might be prevented from reproduction via external forces, however, Meigs renders the obstacles to women's reproduction very differently. Although he briefly flags external forces (the economic times we live in) as playing a role, he ultimately constructs failed reproduction as a consequence of women's agency, through noting that only 'modern' women do not reproduce and lamenting the fact that women 'put off' childbearing. Neither caged nor domesticated, women, unlike monkeys, emerge as 'free' subjects, but bound, importantly, by an obligation to nature. The notion that reproduction is both an obligation and a choice is reiterated when Meigs calls upon doctors to 'teach' and 'urge' women how to have children. Drawing women and monkeys together in these excerpts therefore functions in a number of important ways. First, it attributes subjecthood to both women and monkeys. Secondly, it constructs reproduction as natural and normal for such subjects. Thirdly, it recognises that reproduction among these subjects sometimes fails to occur. Among monkeys, any failure to reproduce is always already a product of *exterior* forces bearing down upon them, whereas women's failure to reproduce is always already an act of free will emerging from *within*. In this way, Meigs' account materialises agency as a 'localisable attribution', after Barad (2007: 217) and then distributes it unevenly as between women and monkeys. Here, like Latour's door-stopper, the monkeys are agentive, playing a vital part in the production of women's subjectivity and agency, mainly through their own reproductive habits.

Insofar as endometriosis emerges as associated with the failure to reproduce, Meigs' account performs the disease as a product of women's inappropriate and unnatural exercise of agency. Interestingly, this account of the human female subject is only partially consistent with the way in which binaries are typically thought to align. More often than not, women are symbolically positioned as passive, rather than active, choosing subjects. The Meigs account operates, therefore, to produce a particular version of the human/nonhuman binary in which agency is distributed in ways that disrupt normative understandings of female subjects. But this works to troubling effect, because in configuring women as agents, women's actions and choices seem to have an important place in materialising the nascent epidemic. This, of course, produces women as culpable in the development of the epidemic and renders them as a legitimate target for biomedical intervention. But more about that later.

The monkeys in the Ballweg account are dealt with somewhat differently and do not, for example, feature as centrally as Meigs' monkeys. Although it was hailed as a major scientific breakthrough, the discovery of endometriosis among the monkey colony was apparently 'incidental'. One could be forgiven for assuming that the monkeys played little or no part in generating the breakthrough; indeed, most accounts of the Rier study position the scientists and/or Ballweg centrally, with the colony thrust out to the periphery. Such positioning depends upon the monkeys being ascribed a largely 'passive' function in the scientific enterprise. Again, this interpretation depends upon a realist understanding of the world and a set of assumptions about subjects, agency and binaries, among other things. Unlike Casper's foetuses, monkeys do not seem to be ascribed any subjecthood or agency at all. The denial of subjectivity and agency to the monkeys may be founded upon a set of assumptions about medical research and the roles of the subjects and objects involved. As a research cohort, monkeys are merely the recipients of scientific knowledge and expertise, with little or no competency or skill of their own. I want to briefly experiment with what might happen if we do attribute them subjectivity, however. Following both Casper and Latour, I want to argue that far from being merely inert, lifeless objects upon which the scientific skill and expertise of physicians such as Rier are brought to bear, the Ballweg monkeys are subjects who have actively participated in the constitution of endometriosis and, by extension, the epidemic. To borrow a phrase employed by Nicole Vitellone (2011: 201) in her work on injecting drug use, there is no reason to think of these monkeys as anything other than 'alive to the event at hand', or as having a productive function in the materialisation of the disease and the epidemic. If we remain open to the possibility that monkeys are actors just as much as scientists, it becomes possible to recognise the competency and functionality of both groups in the emergence of the dioxin proposition and more. (This may or may not be something we could call 'agency'). In any case, this opens up the question of precisely what the monkeys might be performing in the context of the experiment/ laboratory. There are several possibilities.

The monkeys are, to be sure, performing endometriosis, both materially and discursively. But the materialisation of endometriosis following dioxin exposure works in at least two further ways. First, it operates to produce the inside/ outside dichotomy that I noted earlier – a division enfolded throughout (and simultaneously shaping) the disease. Secondly, it does something we haven't seen up until this point in endometriosis medicine: it enacts a class of substances (dioxins) as inherently distinct from nature/the natural. How is this split between nature and culture achieved? If we look closely at the language used, we can see that this takes place through a series of movements: first, through the articulation of food, water and air as elements of nature, then through the classification of chemicals that circulate through any or all of these as separate and distinct. The designation of 'xeno' to these substances (as with xeno-oestrogen) is also telling, for it automatically marks them as distinct and foreign. These substances emerge as artificial – a form of 'otherness' that is exterior to the natural world. This apparent division between nature and culture is performed and reiterated through each and every additional articulation – however such articulations take place –

in which those chemicals are described as something other than food, water and air (i.e. as something other than the natural). There is a sense in which dialogues about endometriosis as environmental disease automatically produce certain chemicals as always already artificial, so that the dangerous nature of them is, or should be, self-evident. That said, some writers have gone to considerable efforts to illustrate why these substances are likely to be harmful, and in so doing, frequently draw upon notions of the natural body at risk from pollution, penetration and propagation. Chemicals are enacted as inherently unnatural and risky – a contaminant by virtue of their (seemingly prior and artificial) form.

Before I move on, I want to say something briefly on the question of monkeys and agency within the milieu of experimental animal research. There is, I believe, an important sense in which it is problematic, ethically and politically, to talk about animals as 'having' agency or being active in the constitution of phenomena via an experiment. There can be little doubt that although the monkeys have produced the disease/epidemic with those scientists, apparatuses, dioxins etc. that together form the experiment-laboratory, there are limits to the way their agency can be drawn. The monkeys have not, for instance, chosen to participate in these experiments, nor asked to be caged and/or administered large doses of dioxin. There is also no method by which they can consent – rather, members of a human research ethics committee are likely to have done so 'for' them, therein shaping the formations of agency as and between the 'humans' and the 'monkeys'. Also, of course, the dioxin experiments are said to have caused many monkeys to develop severe endometriosis and in at least two instances, this resulted in death. So what might we take from this? Among other things, I think this neatly demonstrates Karen Barad's point mentioned earlier, regarding the framing of referents and the formation and attribution of agency. It doesn't do, that is, to make assumptions about what agency looks like (something that can be assigned, characterised by free will, the ability to consent, the capacity to act upon the world, etc.) before we examine a given phenomenon. Agency, instead, *circulates* in various ways, with such arrangements always formulated as specific to and a product of the phenomena in question. This observation, I argue, can be understood as yet another one of the enactments to emerge through Rier's monkeys and my final observation, therefore, about what the monkeys, as actors, *do*. They are agentive in some respects (materialising disease and epidemic as participants in the experiment) but not in others (it is not an experiment of their choosing). They remind us that agency has multiple meanings and is always already a specific and locally enacted phenomenon, the formation and circulation of which is neither stable nor prior to the social relations within which it is formed.

2. Chaos, Order, Modernity and Tradition

Accounts from medical research and advocacy also work to materialise important links between modernity and tradition, chaos and order. My use of the terms 'modern' or 'modernity' may have a tendency to confuse in this context, especially given the current use and usages of these terms in some sectors of academia (I am thinking, specifically, about sociology). In recent years, for instance, sociologists have engaged in a set of vigorous debates about what it means to speak about the 'modern' or 'modernity'. Among other things, these debates have explored the best way to describe the current 'phase' of modernity and the conditions within which we live. In this respect, terms such as 'late', 'high' and 'liquid' modernity are regularly deployed and contested (see, for example, Bauman 2000; Beck 1992; Giddens 1991). For the purposes of the discussion I am having here, I want to be clear that I do not intend to engage with any of these issues, nor with the question of which of these terms more 'accurately' describes the conditions of existence for twenty-first century subjects. Instead, I approach both 'modernity' and 'the modern' as fluid concepts within the context of endometriosis research and advocacy. The meanings attributed to the 'modern', I argue, are both changing and changeable, the form and content of which is constituted through various material-discursive relations, including the work of researchers and advocates. The modern, in short, is *performed* in discourses of medical research and advocacy in ways that may bear little resemblance to the way that the 'modern' and/or 'modernity' is performed in academic debates about contemporary life. Bearing in mind, then, that I do not consider 'modernity' to possess any meaning prior to its enactment through biomedicine, health policy and practice, self-help movements and popular media, I want to argue that the accounts from research and advocacy that I examine here materialise the modern and make the modern in diverse but interrelated ways.

The accounts from Meigs and Ballweg materialise modernity as characterised by various processes, including, most notably, declining reproduction and the spread of chemicals. In Meigs' writings, modernity also has a series of race and class-based features of considerable significance. We will recall that in his published works, he was not simply concerned that women's reproduction was falling and that endometriosis was on the rise, but that a fall in reproduction was taking place at an alarming rate among white and well-educated women – the group that he described, in 1950, as 'our people'. Meigs' concerns with race, class and reproduction coincided with a period in American history, from around the turn of the twentieth century and beyond, in which African–American and European immigrants were reproducing at a higher rate than white, 'Anglo–Saxon' Protestants (Ehrenreich and English 1978: 134). A central concern amongst politicians and medical experts at the time was that America might witness a kind of 'race suicide' (Ehrenreich and English 1978: 135) as a consequence of those reproductive habits and patterns. Whatever the reasons for the falling rates of reproduction amongst white 'Anglo–Saxon' Protestants, experts and politicians believed the problem to be women: they were not doing their 'duty' (Ehrenreich and English 1978: 135). Meigs' work to raise awareness of the condition amongst his fellow physicians appeared driven, at least partly, by concerns about this impending race-based, class-based suicide. Importantly, as I have already noted, Meigs understood these changes to be a uniquely 'modern' phenomenon – a feature, that is, of modernity as he understood it. Meigs' conceptualisation of tradition is therefore one in which race and class are ordered in a very particular way. Moreover, modernity for Meigs is characterised by 'modern' women's turn away from their traditional childbearing role. For Meigs, then, endometriosis is both the origin and end product of modernity in 'crisis', a decline in tradition and the materialisation of modernity gone awry.

In the Ballweg account, human exposure to dioxins is constructed as a relatively recent phenomenon, and in this sense, as a new, novel, and distinctly 'modern' threat. In this way, the monkeys of the dioxin studies perform dioxins as a modern phenomenon, and the modern as unnatural.[6] Insofar as endometriosis is also acknowledged to be a serious disease, the modern 'itself' emerges as a source of palpable harm. Interestingly, there are several paradoxical dimensions to this crisis. In the Ballweg account, xeno-oestrogens, for example, figure as dangerous, foreign, unnatural and an exemplar of modernity gone awry when they are ingested by women. Xeno-oestrogens are also administered as a form of medical treatment, however, because hormonal treatment is a central component of the biomedical approach to treating the disease. Medical treatments rarely figure as similarly unnatural, dangerous and foreign, however. This is interesting, especially because the stated aim of much biomedical treatment for women with endometriosis is usually the cessation of menstruation, a practice that could be read as a kind of 'tampering with nature'. Also, the administration of these hormones is usually understood to produce a series of uncomfortable, debilitating and sometimes permanent side effects for women. If both xeno-oestrogen and hormonal therapies are understood – in the biomedical imaginary, at least – to manipulate the 'normal' or 'natural' body through the disruption of hormones, why are the former positioned as inherently threatening, unnatural and chaotic, while the latter are not? And what does this tell us about nature, culture, modernity and the epidemic?

I suggest that the answers to these questions may lie in the way that both substances are understood to function. As Braidotti (1994) has argued, the meaning and materiality of technologies is not fixed. Technology is often understood as non-threatening and stabilising when, for instance, it is used to aid human

---

6 To be clear, I am not arguing here that constructions of the environment–body connection are uniquely modern or new. As Linda Nash (2006) has argued, the problems thought to be posed by pesticides in the twentieth century were not the catalyst for the emergence of new claims of the relationship between health and environment; instead, they permitted a reconnection with traditional ecological understandings of the relationships between disease and place. Nash (2006: 6) argues that the conception of the body as separate from its environment is a uniquely modernist one and that the neglect of these possible connections is better understood as 'a brief period of modernist amnesia'. My interest is less in these historical understandings than in the way that the modern is constituted in the Ballweg account. It is perhaps of added interest (and significance) that Ballweg treats the environment-body connection as if it is new, thereby producing it as a distinctly novel phenomenon.

reproduction, in part because the promotion and achievement of reproduction is considered a worthwhile aim. On the other hand, technologies that are performed as incompatible with such aims often figure as sinister. Dioxins, as I have explained, are often described as having an inherently *disruptive* potential, which may include, for example, inhibiting the body's capacity to identify endometrial tissue growing in places where it is not 'supposed' to be. Importantly, dioxin is a substance that has been written about elsewhere, and is said to be centrally implicated in compromising women's fertility – not just via endometriosis. In the book *Our Stolen Future*, for example, Colborn, Dumanoski and Myers (1996) raise concerns about the possibility that various chemicals in the environment have the effect of being 'hormone-disrupting'. Although medications administered to women with endometriosis are also described as 'hormone-disrupting', there seems to be less concern, presumably because medical treatment is understood to disrupt hormones in a way that will ultimately lead to the *restoration* of women's fertility, rather than the *decline* of it. In this sense, the presumed and intended 'effects' of these substances bears crucially upon how those same substances are understood to operate, so that only one of the two emerges as hazardous and as implicated in the burgeoning epidemic. To the extent that medications are thought to potentially further women's reproductive capacities, they become aligned to the restoration of tradition, order and the natural body, all of which are produced, as we know, as inherently valuable and desirable. At the same time, chemicals that are thought to impact on reproduction figure as symbolic and material sources of abnormality and chaos. In saying this, I do not mean to argue for a reading of these substances that denies their materiality entirely. Indeed, the point is that the material and discursive here work to co-constitute one another, circulating back through one another in the making of the epidemic. The existence of medication that may help to restore women's health and fertility thus works to reinforce the abject status of dioxins, and all of those binaries with which these substances have become symbolically aligned.

Conclusions

In accounts from medical research and advocacy, endometriosis is performed as an emergent and distinctly 'modern' epidemic in which nature/culture, human/ nonhuman and modernity/tradition figure as being symbolically and literally at war with each other, respectively. The epidemic is, in every sense, an epidemic of the modern: it is an epidemic 'caused' by modernity and an epidemic of modernity, an epidemic that symbolises the modern at the same time as it materialises it. This is an interesting phenomenon, not in the least because modernity is so often understood as a signifier for progress, and progress as inherently positive and desirable. Although endometriosis appears to pose a symbolic challenge to this taken-for-granted idea, appearing as a possible counterpoint to dominant discourses on the merits of modernity, the disease is best understood as a symbol for the value of *ordered* modernity.

The analysis I have undertaken in this chapter lays bare the fluidity, dynamism and malleability of binary categories, whilst also seeking to disrupt and challenge them. This also includes the binary logic of reality/representation, where texts and articulations (like the ones I have examined in this chapter) are understood to merely depict that which already exists (a reality 'out there') instead of being fundamentally implicated in the making of it.[7] Although, as I have already argued, binaries are neither pre-existing nor ontologically stable, the specificities of these binaries and their symbolic and material associations are characterised by both continuity and flux. This point is most apparent when we consider what coheres as and between the two accounts I have considered, and what does not. In the writings of Meigs, endometriosis was primarily enacted as a disease that afflicted white women who delayed childbearing. A 'natural body' was primarily drawn as one in which reproduction occurs (and frequently). Failure to reproduce was effected as a kind of artifice, and as abnormal, as well as at odds with 'tradition'. In this example, the two main threats to the sanctity and ontological security of the natural body are women themselves and external pressures of the period (such as the economy), although the emphasis was almost exclusively on women's disordered choices. In the dioxin studies, the 'natural' body emerges as something different. It is primarily performed as an enclosed, clean and pure entity, whose purity is marked by its lack of association with certain kinds of 'foreign' substances. In this instance, Ballweg's 'natural' body and the threats posed to it are more closely aligned with Margrit Shildrick's concept of the 'leaky body' (1997). According to Shildrick, biomedicine and bioethics frequently construct women's bodies as inherently permeable and 'leaky'. In contrast, the ideal and 'natural' (masculine) body is one that is bounded, secure, and stable – and in this sense, a symbol of purity and order. As a consequence, to the extent that women's bodies might 'leak' or expose the transgression of boundaries, women represent a symbolic and material threat to order. The dioxin studies reflect and reproduce these concerns, producing threats to the bounded, natural body as a source of immense political and ethical concern. In so doing, that account, like Meigs' before it, produces women with endometriosis as a source of immense political and ethical concern.

Importantly, as these examples show, the ideas mobilised in the two accounts I have explored here point to differing but interrelated concerns about what natural bodies should look like, as well as how such bodies should function. Although there are obvious differences in the way both accounts construct the 'natural body', each example touches upon and reproduces a set of gendered concerns about bodies. There is, therefore, a sense of both continuity and flux in these accounts, with the natural body cohering in each example as one that is free from 'artifice' – it is just that what constitutes such artifice differs considerably. As I noted at the outset

---

7   For more, see Fraser and Seear (2011: 46–7).

of this chapter, the two examples I chose for analysis here emerge somewhere between 30 and 50 years apart, so it is not unexpected to imagine that they will diverge in some ways. The fact that these accounts cohere in important ways is perhaps even more interesting. This continuity demonstrates that endometriosis coheres across time, even though it is enacted multiply by different advocates, as a relatively 'new' disease (cf. Nezhat, Nezhat and Nezhat 2012) fundamentally preoccupied with the modern and with the need to contain, control and manage it. Although I have focused on two examples from medical research and advocacy here, it is possible that other examples may materialise their own versions of the 'natural' body as well, and that these versions may change in future, as new thinking about the disease and the epidemic emerge.

In *AIDS and the Body Politic*, with which I opened this chapter, Waldby argued that the war on a virus or disease that is the subject of an epidemic is also always a war on the people who suffer from that disease. She points out that declarations of war 'allow the deployment of legitimate violence, and the suspension of normal civil rights', so that people with the disease often find themselves caught up in various strategies of violence, 'cast in terms of preventative, therapeutic or diagnostic practices' (1996: 4). Drawing upon the work of Linda Singer (1993) and Michel Foucault (1978, 1997), Waldby goes on to argue that even greater forms of regulation and self-governance are considered legitimate in the context of HIV/AIDS because it is both an epidemic (war) and a *sexual* epidemic, where the very capacity of humankind to reproduce itself is understood to be placed at risk. This 'sharpens' the war at hand, as:

> Under conditions of sexual epidemic each sex and sexual orientation becomes a disease threat to the other, exacerbating existing tensions between masculinity and femininity, heterosexuality and homosexuality. (1996: 8)

To some extent, the endometriosis epidemic is also a sexual epidemic, insofar as the disease is understood to represent a major threat to the fertility of women. Some estimates, as I noted at the outset of this book, put the global incidence at 200 million, or the prevalence as high as 10 per cent of menstruating women, and rising. Although I would not want to conflate endometriosis with infertility (for reasons that will become clearer as the book unfolds), the possible impact of the disease on the reproducibility of humanity is often cited – especially by health advocates – as a cause for alarm. In this way, the endometriosis epidemic is performed as a crisis point, where panics around sexuality, reproduction and modernity surface and coalesce.

For all of these reasons, women with endometriosis simultaneously embody and enact the crisis of the modern, emerging as sources of horror: disordered, chaotic and inherently threatening. Insofar as women with endometriosis also straddle several key dualisms, they are 'cyborgs' (Haraway 1991, 1985) – hybrid organisms that subvert preconceptions about the inherent and essential stability of distinctions between nature, culture, artifice, and the like. The need to detect, treat and 'cure' these subversives therefore emerges as virtually self-evident. The bodies of women with the disease become the surfaces upon which a further set of battles – to contain the abject subject and preserve human fertility – will be played out. Attempts to engage with patients and/or treat the disease must therefore be understood as borne within and bearing upon these various politically, racially, gendered and sexually charged configurations. One of the key concerns of this book, then, is with the ways that women with endometriosis figure as the symbolic and literal manifestations of the modern – or, more precisely, the *hazardous aspects of modernity*. Attempts to manage the epidemic are at least partly a means through which the disordered aspects of modernity 'itself' – however these are constituted – might be governed. This has potentially enormous ramifications for the lived experiences of women who live with endometriosis, as we will see in the chapters that follow.

Chapter 2
The Disease of Theories:
On the Function of Medical Hypotheses

Endometriosis is "the disease of theories".

(Chandler 2000)

As I explained in the Introduction, endometriosis has been variously described as 'puzzling' (Berbic and Fraser 2011; Ballweg 2003d), an 'enigma' (Thomas 1993), 'mysterious' (Holloway 1994), 'complex' (Gao et al. 2006), 'elusive' (Quinn 2009) and 'enigmas wrapped in riddles' (Jaffe 2004: xv). Uncertain in its aetiology, as well as its 'effect', and widely considered to be a complex and mysterious disease, endometriosis has been referred to as 'the disease of theories' (Chandler 2000). This is because in the 150 years since its 'discovery', the cause of endometriosis has been the subject of constant speculation. The aetiology and pathogenesis of the disease remain largely unknown, there is a lack of consensus as to how to treat the condition and a cure remains elusive. Indeed, as Sloan (1947: 27) argued more than 65 years ago:

> No condition in the field of gynecology exhibits such a variety of manifestations as does endometriosis. No other condition has in consequence been so prolific of speculation and theory to explain it.

Today, speculation and theory are still a constant of the condition. The prevalence of disease theories in relation to any disease might be considered as largely unexceptional. After all, theories are ubiquitous in contemporary biomedicine, whether they pertain to the causes of a disease or syndrome, the conditions under which a virus may spread, debates about the gold standards for treatment of any given disease, or mooted preventative strategies for avoiding disease risks. Vast textbooks and library shelves are dedicated to musings on all of these things and more, with an array of diseases, viruses and syndromes involved. So, it might be said, the 'mere' existence of theories in relation to any disease state is unremarkable. But in this chapter I argue that the 'mere' existence of theories in relation to any disease – but especially endometriosis – *is* remarkable. In what follows, I argue that the articulation and deployment of disease theories is significant because *theories enact the world*. Disease theories are a fundamental part of the process by which a set of relations between medicine, the subject and disease are produced and reproduced. As well as this, theories have a doubly significant role to play in diseases of uncertain aetiology, for reasons I will explore.

This chapter explores two main questions. First: what can we learn from the 'mere' existence of theories about endometriosis? I use the word 'mere' very intentionally here, and primarily as a way of reminding the reader of the common assumption that the simple presence of theories in biomedicine is neither remarkable nor significant, beyond their utility for the field itself. (For ease, I will refrain from using inverted commas from this point on, although all references to the 'mere' existence of theories should be read with this caveat in mind). The insistence on and persistence with theorising in any field, but especially, I will argue, medicine, is a practice with which we need to grapple more critically. This is because, as I have already suggested, *theories do things*. This occurs by virtue of their mere articulation, but also through the specific content of the theories themselves. The second question that this chapter addresses is: how does medicine handle the preponderance of theories with regards endometriosis? This is an important question for reasons that will become apparent, including, most notably, the fact that the production and proliferation of theories threatens on the face of it to undermine conventional perceptions of medicine as coherent, ordered and ordering, unified and rational. What is the significance of medicine's apparent failure to come to grips with endometriosis, to understand the mechanisms of the disease, including its aetiology, and to find a cure? These questions are explored through an analysis of medical and scientific literature in which theories about the disease are articulated, reproduced, debated and reviewed.[1] The central argument I advance is a simple one: that theories participate in the enactment of the world. This is despite the fact that theory, 'materiality' and 'reality' are ordinarily portrayed as separate 'things', or as ontologically disconnected and separate. I also argue that the production and deployment of theory is a fundamental part of the process by which medicine performs itself as heroic. In this sense, disease theorisations are thoroughly political, and an under-examined component of disease ontics more broadly. In the next sections, I begin with a brief introduction to disease theories in the endometriosis literature. After this, I examine parallels between work on decision making more broadly, especially as explored by John Law (2002), and

---

1   The analysis that I undertake in this chapter emerges out of an initial (larger) study of the history of endometriosis medicine since 1860. In that study, I conducted searches through a range of common search engines – such as PubMed and Google Scholar – for medical and scientific literature regarding the history, origins, aetiology and treatment of the disease. When a search is conducted in Google Scholar (as of April 2013), almost 35,000 documents are returned. My initial searches were therefore refined so that studies on aetiology, treatment and the history of the disease were returned. In my initial review of these materials it was quickly established that the production and deployment of disease theories was a key feature of the gynaecological literature. With this in mind, then, I isolated medical texts and papers published on the nature, history and origins of the disease between 1990 and 2013. For this chapter, I focused primarily on papers and texts in which disease theories were articulated, debated, reviewed and discussed. These studies were qualitatively analysed using a form of discourse analysis that I describe in more detail in Seear (2009a).

the process of articulating and debating disease theories. I consider how Law understands the articulation of options – and the process of making decisions about those options – within the context of policy making, after which I examine how these ideas might be usefully applied – or not – to the study of disease theorisation. After this, I apply some of these ideas to an analysis of endometriosis medicine and conclude with a consideration of what this means for the disease more broadly.

Processes of Deliberation

Decision-making has been the subject of considerable academic interest over the last few decades, with interest from fields as diverse as sociology, management, medicine, law and economics (March 1994). Although the approach varies depending on the specific field involved, the process of making and implementing decisions is often understood as a means by which power is exercised. So, as March (1994: 141–2) explains, for example, power is central to accounts of decision-making in several ways:

> Although the assumption can be misleading, most theories of decision making assume that power is desired, that each individual wants to have decisions made that are consistent with his or her preferences and identities.

Although there are different models of decision-making and power, publics often assume that powerful people get what they want, and that one way this might be achieved is through influencing how, which and what decisions are made (March 1994). Such approaches often assume, of course, that power is 'possessed' by some individuals and imposed upon others, a notion that has been thoroughly critiqued by Michel Foucault in his work on discipline, government and power (e.g. Foucault 1980a, 1980b, 1980c, 1977). In recent years, scholars adopting a broadly Foucauldian approach have moved away from this understanding of power, eschewing assumptions about how power vests and circulates. These matters are discussed more fully in chapters three and five, but for the present time it is enough to say that new approaches have emerged in recent years, some of which are influenced by Foucault. The approach that John Law (2002) takes differs again, in that although he is concerned with the ways in which decision-making might be understood as a form of power, he is also concerned with other instances of what decision-making might do. As we will see, Law argues that questions about decision making – including how the need for deliberation is enacted – are crucial, not only because decision making might have a relationship with power, but because it bears in important ways on ontology.

Law's analysis of decision-making is unconventional in many respects. He sets out to consider settings where we might take for granted the notion that decisions are – or need to be – made, seeking to instead understand how the *obligation* to deliberate is itself brought into being. Law also wants us to think more critically about some of the implications of enacting deliberative processes – what deliberation does, achieves, performs or makes in the world. Taking the realm of Politics – with a capital P – as his focus, Law considers these issues using a case study from the failed TSR2 project. He argues that much can be learnt from attending to a range of documents about the decision to cancel the aircraft, including, for example, the diaries, notes and retrospective accounts of various stakeholders reporting on exactly 'what happened'. His starting point is that the documents he examines are 'a performance and not simply a description' of historic events. These accounts intervene in the aircraft, as well as Politics, with implications for agency, power, ethics and ontology. Starting with accounts of the project's cancellation, Law finds that key stakeholders typically refer to a list of possibilities for the future of the project (to proceed with the aircraft's construction, to cancel the aircraft's development, to cancel it and buy an alternative set of planes, and so on). What this does is produce the cancellation of the project as the outcome of a deliberative process, where that process is enacted via the narrative rather than simply described. The need for deliberation is achieved by positing the project as a set of options (to cancel, to proceed, etc.). In this sense, Law argues,

> Decision making tends to perform itself as the cockpit of difference. It is where, as it were, different options are brought together and focused. (2002: 150)

In the examples that Law attends to, the production of a set of options not only performs an obligation to deliberate, but works to produce what he calls 'a great divide between reality and fantasy' (2002: 147). Crucially,

> None of the exhibits [regarding the project's cancellation] actually says anything about this, presumably because there is no need to. But look, nonetheless, at the way this is done. For instance, all the exhibits take it for granted that the possibilities on offer are *mutually exclusive*, that they are indeed just that, "options" – which means that decision makers need to make a choice between possible scenarios, with the possibility of one, but only one, future reality. Thus the need for "hard choices" is performed for, and by, the British cabinet, and the possibility of what the poststructuralists sometimes call "undecidability" disappears ... Pursuing more than one option is thus performed as a fantasy. (2002: 147)

When options are set out in this way, the need to deliberate becomes both necessary and self-evident. It would not do, that is, to simply list a series of options pertaining to a particular policy issue without also making a *choice* about them.

According to Michael Callon (1986), the positing of options and the process of making decisions about those options always already functions to produce a knowing subject. This is because when options are articulated, someone needs to serve as the subject through whom the options must pass. The knowing subject (or 'decision maker') emerges as the 'obligatory point of passage' for assessing the specific options concerned, emerging as the key figure for delineating between fantasy and reality. A similar argument is made by Bruno Latour in his work on visualisation and cognition, where he develops the notion of a 'centre for calculation'. As Latour (1986: 29) explains:

> Money per se is certainly not the universal standard looked for by Marx and other economists. This qualification should be granted to centers of calculation and to the peculiarity of written traces which makes rapid translation between one medium and another possible. Many efforts have been made to link the history of science with the history of capitalism, and many efforts have been made to describe the scientist as a capitalist. All these efforts (including mine – Latour and Woolgar, 1979: chap. 5; Latour 1984a) were doomed from the start, since they took for granted a division between mental and material factors, an artifact of our ignorance of inscriptions. There is not a history of engineers, then a history of capitalists, then one of scientists, then one of mathematicians, then one of economists. Rather, there is a single history of these centers of calculation. It is not only because they look exclusively at maps, account books, drawings, legal texts and files, that cartographers, merchants, engineers, jurists and civil servants get the edge on all the others. It is because all these inscriptions can be superimposed, reshuffled, recombined, and summarized, and that totally new phenomena emerge, hidden from the other people from whom all these inscriptions have been exacted.

Following Latour, Law (2002) argues that accounts of the TSR2 aircraft work to produce politicians as the centre for calculation – or the obligatory point of passage – through whom large and difficult decisions will be made. As well as performing reality and fantasy, then, decision-making renders politicians as 'big' and 'important' (2002: 160). The production of decision-makers as both 'big' and 'important' is an 'effect' of the articulation of options and the production of options as mutually exclusive. Importantly, decision-makers emerge as the arbiters of truth, insofar as decision-making is performed as a method for accessing reality (where 'reality' itself is also enacted). The point that Law wants to make here is that although we might think of politicians and other notable decision-makers (such as judges) as always already big, important, powerful and wise, the constitution of such subjects is in fact an *achievement*. The omnipotent decision maker is an enactment materialised through a series of material-discursive movements including narrative accounts of 'what happened' vis-à-vis a particular phenomenon. This extends even to 'High Politics', as Law calls it, the features of which are neither prior nor fixed. This is a potentially useful idea for thinking through biomedicine, as we shall see.

Pluralism, Fragmentation, Multiplicity

This leads me on to the question of ontology in Law's work. In his examination of different accounts of the decision to cancel the TSR2 aircraft, Law found overlaps between the versions, as well as differences. There were differences, for example, in the number of 'options' facing politicians, and the nature of those options sometimes differed. How might we understand these similarities and differences? The first possibility according to Law is that they are different perspectives on a single decision, but that the differences have been 'smoothed away' (2004: 58) somehow, perhaps because the authors of the accounts forgot what happened, misunderstood how the decision was made, or weren't aware of all of the options. This approach holds that there is 'indeed a single and definite decision ... selected from a single and definite range of options', but that the variation in accounts of the decision is a problem of perspectivalism rather than anything else (2004: 58). In this respect, perspectivalism is both a way of understanding differences in opinion or account, and a means by which singularity is performed out of difference. An alternative explanation can be found in Annemarie Mol's work on multiplicity and involves a very different understanding of what differences might mean:

> This is that the different participants were making *different* decisions, and that they simply thought were making a single decision. Then, somehow or other, they co-ordinated themselves. Imagined themselves to be making the same decision. Displaced the possible differences, kept this apart. Perhaps we might call this "virtual singularity". (Law 2004: 58)

In this case, there are multiple decisions – as opposed to different perspectives on a single decision – but this multiplicity is obscured, as different decisions are made to cohere as if they are one. Difference, as Law (2002) puts it, is 'effaced'. Insofar as decision-making and accounts of decision-making – like anything else – are performative, we see that they may operate to enact the world as multiple, or as singular, as the case may be. As Mol explains in *The Body Multiple* (2002: 83–4), multiplicity should not be confused with pluralism or fragmentation:

> But the ontology that comes with equating what *is* with what is *done* is not of a pluralist kind. The manyfoldedness of objects enacted does not imply their fragmentation. Although atherosclerosis in the hospital comes in different versions, these somehow hold together. A single patient tends to be supplied, if not with a single disease, then at least with a single treatment decision.

I have examined questions around singularity, multiplicity and coherence in my previous work on hepatitis C (Fraser and Seear 2011), with particular interest in the question of how that which is multiple also 'hangs together'. Mol (2002) suggests that objects that are multiple tend to hang together through 'various modes of coordination' that smooth away complexity and mess in favour of order. These modes of coordination include processes of layering, submission, translation, rationalisation and the production of single narratives. Where there is tension, for example, in 'test outcomes … one of them is made to win. A hierarchy is established and the discrepancy between the tests is explained away' (2002: 84). In addition, multiplicity might be regulated in ways that do not result in singularity, such as mutual exclusion, and the creation of composite objects. One example of this may be through the production – using Mol's example – of composite forms of atheroscleroses, such as 'walking-atherosclerosis' and 'pressure-atherosclerosis'. Here, multiplicity is recognised, but in such a way that medicine is still made to 'work'. As these examples reveal, the enactment of objects as multiple and/or singular is a hugely significant process, especially insofar as they often perform and sustain a neat and ordered account of the workings of a given field, like Politics.

Endometriosis, Theory, Multiplicity and Mess

It seems to me that the ideas I have explored above can usefully be extended to other areas of interest in which the requirement to deliberate is materialised, and where variation or difference can also be found. Mess, difference, singularity, multiplicity, decision-making and obligatory points of passage can be found in a range of fields, including medical knowledge and practice. These ideas are especially relevant to the study of endometriosis for a number of reasons. For example, as I have already noted, the endometriosis medical literature is dominated by a plethora of disease theories. These include theories about the disease pathogenesis and the characteristics of its subjects. The articulation of disease theories, like the TSR2 project, produces an obligation for examination, deliberation and decisions to be made. What is the 'disease' in question? Is it one object or two? How might we understand the origins and mechanisms of the disease/s? What theories are available to us? Do the theories overlap in some way? Are there similarities or differences? How do we make choices between them? Do we even need to? Are they merely different perspectives on a single disease, or multiple perspectives on multiple diseases? How is this multiplicity handled? Where processes of coordination leading to virtual singularity can be found, what can we take from them? What are the implications of the means by which endometriosis is made to cohere – or not?

Writing about the rise of causal concepts of disease in the history of medicine, K. Codell Carter (2003: 106) explains the function of disease theories in this way:

> The purposes of any scientific theory are explanation and control. In a theory of disease, achieving either purpose requires universal necessary causes, and such causes depend on etiological characterizations. But etiological characterizations are possible only if the causes in terms of which different diseases are defined

> are themselves distinct. Thus, the formulation of etiological definitions (and
> hence the adequacy of any theory of disease) requires distinguishability.

This seems to me to represent an explicit acknowledgement of the interconnectedness of medical epistemologies (in the form of disease hypotheses) and ontologies. Although Carter speaks of the need for 'distinguishability' in terms of aetiological characterisations, disease hypotheses also depend upon distinguishability as between disease *objects* – a seemingly obvious point, perhaps, but one that might easily be lost. In this respect, disease hypotheses and diseases 'themselves' have a potentially mutually co-constitutive relationship. It would make little sense, that is, to produce hypotheses about the aetiology of a 'disease' without that disease being distinct or distinguishable from other diseases. In this way, the mere articulation of theories about aetiology both necessitates and enacts diseases as distinct. The question then becomes whether diseases are enacted as singular or as multiple, how singularity and multiplicity are achieved and why all of this might matter.

These questions have added interest in the case of endometriosis. Unlike Law, I am not here dealing with an historical artifact about which a major decision has already been made. The novel dimension of Law's case study was that the decision to cancel the project had already been made, so that Law was able to examine – with the benefit of hindsight – numerous extant accounts of an historical decision to see how that decision was understood, coordinated, made coherent and so on. Decisions in the field of endometriosis medicine have already been made, of course, and are continually being made, but there remains a lack of scientific consensus about extant medical hypotheses. Endometriosis is a 'live' disease, the subject of ongoing contest and significant debate – as I flagged briefly in the Introduction – and represents a thoroughly different and unique case study. There is a certain messiness about the disease that complicates things. In addition, the medical literature is punctuated not only by theories about the disease, but by additional commentaries on those theories (including the overall 'state' of medical knowledge). Literature of this kind provides a means for understanding how medicine understands – and manages – itself. Like those retrospective accounts of the TSR2 decision that enact High Politics as 'big' and 'important', medical literature may function in a similar way, especially where accounts offer an appraisal of medical theories. Endometriosis literature is replete with self-reflexive accounts and analyses of this kind; accounts which represent yet another means by which the uncertainty and messiness of medical knowledge and practice is handled, coordinated and made to cohere (or not).

As we will see, these questions are not of mere academic interest, but have major implications for how we understand the ontics of diseases – like endometriosis – that are also thoroughly 'messy' objects. Even if medicine emerges as the obligatory point of passage through the production and deployment of disease theories, what might we take from the continued uncertain aetiology of the disease? Is it possible, for example, that medicine is produced as both big and important, as the obligatory passage point, and a source of failure, insofar as no theory has yet been developed to account for the disease, adequately explain its mechanisms, and so on? Is it possible that endometriosis medicine renders only some physicians and scientists as big and important, while those whose hypotheses are discounted emerge as failed subjects by virtue of having got things 'wrong'? These and other questions are examined in the sections to follow. I begin with a broad overview of how disease theories are often summarised within medical literature and some of the implications of this. I then consider questions of difference and coherence in medicine's understanding of the 'disease of theories'.

Endometriosis and Difference

In their broadest sense, theories suggest ways of thinking about the world, and imply, produce and reproduce arrangements between subjects and objects. Theories exclude and privilege some possibilities – whether they be about the origins of the universe, the meaning of existence, the means for living an ethical life, or what it is to be human. When they do this, theories also explicitly or implicitly promote certain possibilities of being, becoming and living in the world. But let us assume for a moment that theories do nothing, beyond, self-evidently, suggesting possibilities and articulating probabilities. Let us begin with a typical example of disease theorising from the medical literature about endometriosis. In Nap's (2012) recent overview of theories on the pathogenesis of endometriosis, it was said:

> Several hypotheses have been put forward to explain the pathogenesis of the disease ... The concepts of *in situ* development, induction, transplantation, and retrograde menstruation are considered as the most important theories ...

A number of theories are then detailed in a small table, with a longer description of the main theories appearing alongside it. These are (2012: 42–4):

In situ *development*
The oldest concept concerning the pathogenesis of endometriosis is based on the assumption that endometriosis develops *in situ* from local tissue ...

Müllerian remnants
In the embryonic phase, the coelomic epithelium gives rise to the müllerian ducts which form the fallopian tubes, the uterine body, the cervix, and the upper part of the vagina. Aberrant differentiation or migration of the müllerian ducts could cause spreading of cells in the migratory pathway of fetal organogenesis across the posterior pelvic floor.

Coelomic metaplasia

The theory of coelomic metaplasia suggests that the germinal epithelium of the ovary and the serosa of the peritoneum can be transformed into endometrium by metaplasia. These metaplastic changes occur secondary to inflammatory processes or hormonal changes …

Induction

The theory of induction may be seen as an extension of the coelomic metaplasia theory, proposing that one or several endogenous, biochemical or immunological factors could induce endometrial differentiation in undifferentiated cells …

Transplantation

The theory of transplantation implies that endometrium is replaced from the uterus to another location inside the body. Different routes of dissemination are involved in the concept of transplantation in the pathogenesis of endometriosis …

Retrograde menstruation

The most popular theory is Sampson's retrograde menstruation theory. Initially, Sampson assumed that endometriotic lesions are seedlings from diseased ovaries. Later on, in 1927, he proposed that endometriosis is the result of the reflux of endometrial fragments through the fallopian tubes during menstruation, with subsequent implantation and growth on and into the peritoneum and the ovary.

Nap's is a fairly typical summary of theories of the disease. Like accounts of the TSR2's cancellation, summaries of this kind produce the underlying mechanisms of endometriosis – and the disease itself – as a set of options from which, it seems, a choice must be made. To borrow a phrase from John Law (2002), the disease is performed as *either this, that or the other*. Although theories about endometriosis are usually positioned as a set of mutually exclusive options, it is also possible for them to figure as a collection of interrelated or overlapping possibilities (i.e. as this, that or the other, or as a bit of this and that, or a combination of that and the other). Where there is a potentially synergistic relation between them (as there is with endometriosis), these are best understood as simply further options. So, the disease might be understood as:

Produced by mechanism A
Produced by mechanism B
Produced by mechanism C
Produced by mechanism D
Produced by A in combination with C
Produced when D acts upon B

And so on. Theories about the disease often include explicit deliberations on the likely 'nature' of the condition. So, for example, theorists who subscribe to Sampson's theory of retrograde menstruation may often refer to it as a 'gynaecological' disease, while others emphasise endometriosis as an 'immunological disorder'. Where the coelomic metaplasia theory is endorsed, endometriosis may also be described as an 'inflammatory' or 'genetic' disorder, or perhaps, some combination of the two.

Although these details are important, I am presently less interested in the specificities of disease theory and/or the tendency to categorise endometriosis as one type of disorder or another, then in what we can take from the articulation of disease options. Most obviously, these formulations are underpinned by an assumption that there is a specific disease entity to which the theories pertain. In this way, medical hypotheses perform endometriosis as a unique and distinct object – as singular, in Mol's terms. On the other hand, theories of what the disease 'is' and/or how it 'works' perform endometriosis as unstable, complex and incoherent through suggesting that the mechanisms of the disease – if not the disease itself – remain unclear. In enacting endometriosis as unstable and uncertain in this way, medicine opens up the possibility that endometriosis may be multiple. Importantly, this also opens up the possibility that medicine itself is non-coherent, lacking in unity, prone to error and irrational, especially where theories continue to be thrown up without resolution. I want to argue that medical literature has a way of resolving these tensions so that difference and uncertainty is regulated in ways that preserve medicine's power. In order to understand how this happens we need to attend more closely to what is going on alongisde the articulation and deployment of disease theories. Through various rhetorical devices and strategies, medicine assigns responsibility for uncertainty to the disease itself, and smooths away complexities. In this sense, medical theories hold both disease and medicine together through a range of material-discursive practices. In the next sections I attend to four specific practices of holding together:

1. The production of the disease as inherently enigmatic;
2. The production of menstrual tissue and blood as evasive;
3. The claim that endometriosis is not a disease at all;
4. The claim that endometriosis is a set of diseases.

The Disease Enigma

The first way that medicine handles uncertainty, variation and its own propensity towards theorising is through the production of what Mol (2002) calls a 'single narrative'. Single narratives are devices that smooth over differences, contradictions and uncertainties so as to avoid non-coherence. In the present case, medical hypotheses are accompanied by depictions of endometriosis as inherently 'enigmatic', 'puzzling', 'mysterious' and so on. The true mechanisms of the disease have also been described as a 'black box' (Evers 2010: xviii), or as being held 'under lock and key' (Nezhat, Nezhat and Nezhat 2012: 58). As I flagged at the start of the chapter, these descriptions of the disease are common. As Evers (2010: xvii) notes, for instance, 'In almost every textbook endometriosis is characterised as *"enigmatic"'*. In this way, the differences we encounter in medical literature are explained away through an overarching narrative in which the disease figures as singularly enigmatic. In so doing, medicine performs the incomprehensibility of the disease as a function of the disease *itself.* This narrative operates to obscure the extent to which medical knowledge and practice might be limited, as it assigns responsibility for ongoing uncertainty to something other than medicine. Importantly, these depictions maintain a commitment to ontological singularity by performing endometriosis as a single disease, while explaining variation and/or difference as effects of the disease's innate characteristics. Although uncertainty and difference are explicitly acknowledged, and not just buried away, they are at the same time rendered insignificant beyond their utility for securing medicine as a still-rational enterprise.

It is no coincidence that depictions of the disease echo traditional representations of women and the feminine, as mysterious, puzzling and enigmatic (e.g. Ussher 2006; Pollock 2003; Irigaray 1985). As Freud (1973) argued in *On Femininity*, for example:

> Throughout human history people have knocked their heads against the riddle
> of the nature of femininity ... Nor will you have escaped worrying over this
> problem – those of you who are men; to those of you who are women this will
> not apply – you are yourselves the problem.

This approach was famously critiqued by Luce Irigaray (1985: 13), who argued that:

> The enigma that is woman will therefore constitute the *target*, the *object*, the
> *stake*, of a masculine discourse, of a debate among men, which would not
> consult her, would not concern her. Which, ultimately, she is not supposed to
> know anything about.

In a similar vein Elizabeth Grosz (1994: 191) has explained that:

> the enigma that Woman has posed for men is an enigma only because the male
> subject has construed itself as the subject par excellence. The way (he fantasizes)
> that Woman differs from him makes her containable within his imagination
> (reduced to his size) but also produces her as a mystery for him to master and
> decipher within safe or unthreatening borders.

In this way, references to endometriosis as enigmatic function as a *metonym* for women and the feminine, and serve to reinforce the notion of women and femininity as inherently perplexing. At the same time, descriptions of the disease and its subjects as inherently mysterious and perplexing function to produce and reproduce men and masculinity as signifiers of the 'truth' and truth seeking. These symbolic alignments between the masculine and truth/truth-seeking, on the one hand, and women/ femininity as perplexing, on the other enacts medicine as the realm of truth. All of these ideas are mutually reinforcing and stabilising, working to produce the mysteries of the disease as a product of the mysterious feminine. In this way, medical uncertainty, non-coherence and difference (whether in terms of the disease object 'itself' or the mechanisms that produce it) emerge as an artefact of the feminine, rather than expressions of shortcomings within medical knowledge and practice.

Evading Capture

As an extension of this, medical literature renders menstrual blood and tissue as having a particularly active and elusive quality that obscures the origins and nature of ongoing uncertainties pertaining to the disease, including differences between disease theories and accounts of what the disease actually 'is'. The best example of this is in medical depictions of 'the most widely accepted' theory of development (Evers 2010; Redwine 2002) for endometriosis, a theory known as 'retrograde' or 'reflux menstruation'. In a 'seminal' (Benagiano and Brosens 2006: 459) 1927 paper, Sampson finalised a detailed hypothesis on the issue of the misplacement of endometrial tissue. This theory, noted earlier, has dominated clinical and scientific approaches to the disease ever since (Benagiano and Brosens 2006: 459) and continues to be the most popular theory of the disease's mechanical processes.[2] Put simply, the reflux theory posits that menstrual blood and cells flow backwards through the fallopian tubes during menstruation and implant throughout the uterus (Benagiano and Brosens 2006: 459). As Nap (2012: 44) explains:

> The reflux menstruation theory is based on the assumption that retrograde menstruation takes place and that viable endometrial tissue reaches the abdominal cavity and implants. These three conditions are the basic principles of the viability of Sampson's theory.

Although retrograde flow was initially thought to be rare (with prevalence likely to be somewhere between 5–15 per cent of women, alongside estimates of the disease) it has since been claimed through several studies that reflux occurs in more than 85–90 per cent of women (e.g. Redwine 2009). So, as Giudice (2010: 2389) explains: 'Although most women have retrograde menstruation, not all women with retrograde menstruation have endometriosis'.

---

2   Although some (for example, Redwine 2002) dispute Sampson's theory.

In spite of this possible flaw in the retrograde hypothesis, Sampson's theory has not been abandoned. It has, however, become a central point of focus in debates about the disease. One effect of this has been a redoubling of efforts to determine exactly why some women go on to develop endometriosis while others do not, when the vast majority of women experience retrograde flow. If most women experience reflux flow, why do only a fraction of them develop the disease? Does tissue carried by blood always implant? How and why might it implant in only some instances? Is it possible that Sampson was wrong and that something else explains the disease? To admit as much now would be to abandon nearly 100 years of thinking on the subject, and the commitment to reflux as central in the development of the disease.

These few questions represent an instance of variance and/or difference within a single disease theory, a different phenomenon to the one I have earlier described, where differences as between theories are found. Medicine manages these tensions through a process of *rationalisation* (Mol 2002), where inconsistencies and impasses in medical knowledge and practice are explained away. In the present case this is achieved through two interrelated discursive moves. First, medicine performs menstruation as an intrinsically *elusive* process, so that, like accounts that perform the disease as an enigma, a degree of instability and uncertainty in medical knowledge is constituted as inherent to the disease. Secondly, menstrual blood and tissue is performed as possessing special abilities and traits; these traits enable the underlying pathogenesis of the disease to repeatedly evade capture. One effect of these discursive manoeuvres is that even if reflux occurs amongst most – or even all – women, the tissue confounds us in some way in some cases, generating uncertainties and unpredictable results. In rationalising problems with disease theory in this way, medicine is conceding – yet again – the limitations of current knowledge and practice. This may or may not be consistent with multiplicity. Whatever is going on, it is menstruation 'itself' that is responsible. I will explain how this happens.

A central component of Sampson's retrograde hypothesis is that viable endometrium is transported in menstrual blood, deposited in other parts of the uterus and somehow 'attaches' itself (Chalmers 1975: 8). This notion – of viable cells 'attaching' themselves to the uterine surface – is often utilised in medical literature. Redwine (2002: 687) describes the theoretical mechanism in this way:

> ... endometriosis occurs as a result of the reflux of menstrual blood out through the fimbriated end of the fallopian tubes, this blood carrying with it viable cells from the endometrial lining which could attach to peritoneal surfaces, proliferate, invade, and become the disease known as endometriosis.

In this account, Redwine attributes a dynamic quality to menstrual blood and endometrial matter – one where blood refluxes upwards and outwards from the fallopian tubes, 'carrying' cells with it. Once beyond the fallopian tubes, viable cells transported in the blood 'attach' to surfaces, where they 'proliferate' and 'invade' the surrounding surfaces. In this account, menstrual blood emerges as active, dynamic and vital. In another example, Evers (2010: xviii) also performs menstrual blood and tissue as lively, insofar as refluxed endometrium 'activates' the immune system and then 'elicits an inflammatory response'. On the other hand, the uterine cavity is constituted as both prone to invasion and torpid in the face of it. Metaphorical depictions of endometrial tissue as an invader of the womb have continued in more recent depictions of how the disease 'works' (for example, Brosens and Brosens 2000: 161). Evers' (1996: 352) description of the mechanism of implantation is a useful illustration of this, and begins to invoke further, more complex metaphors, positioning the womb as being 'at war' with endometrial tissue:

> Fragments of functional endometrium reflux through the Fallopian tubes and reach the, essentially hostile, environment of the peritoneal cavity. Proteolytic activity, activated macrophages, and natural killer cells all combine to degrade and digest the regurgitated tissue fragments. Single cells escaping this defence mechanism loose their adhesive properties and thus cannot implant. Occasionally whole fragments of endometrial tissue succeed in evading the peritoneal defence lines, perhaps by their sheer number, perhaps by an intrinsic defect in the defence mechanism.

The most striking feature of this account is the way in which the 'body' surfaces as fragmented. It is akin to a series of component parts, with one part (the peritoneal cavity) emerging as a 'hostile environment'. Through the mobilisation of military metaphors, the pelvis emerges as a battle zone, where 'killer' cells, and 'fragments' of endometrial tissue – like enemies in battle – find ways to evade the 'lines' of defence. According to Birnbaum and Cummings (2002: 15), endometriosis involves the endometrial cells being:

> ... able to attach to organs and/or tissues on which they have landed. Once attached, the endometrial cells may be able to invade the underlying tissue, leading to deep lesions.

The idea of the pelvis being invaded by tissues that have 'landed' on the surface has more than a hint of science fiction about it. But it is the pelvis' war with dispersed endometrial tissue – deployed via notions of evasion and capture – that dominates medical literature on the hypothesis, as well as reviews on the viability of the theory. As Rose (2005: 14) argues, for example:

> Normally, natural killer (NK) cells would remove refluxed menstrual debris from the peritoneal cavity ... It is unclear whether these NK cells in endometriosis patients are "faulty" (i.e. unable to recognize the endometrial cells and thereby destroy them), or whether the endometrial cells have a special ability to prevent recognition by NK cells.

In this account, through some as yet unexplained process, endometrial cells may have a *special* capacity to camouflage themselves and evade capture. The cells are enemy combatants; although they should be recognised as foreign and destroyed, through their cunning and connivance, they somehow manage to survive and to thrive. Through these accounts, the difficulties thrown up by the retrograde menstruation hypothesis are resolved in a way that reconciles difference and mess while preserving two seemingly inconsistent possibilities – that retrograde flow occurs amongst most (or all) women and is implicated in the disease's development, yet only a fraction of women go on to develop the disease. All of this is, naturally, possible, and I do not mean to suggest otherwise in my account of the literature. Instead, I am interested in the way in which medicine reconciles these inconsistencies and tensions through processes of rationalisation which include the possibility of additional factors being implicated in the disease. Importantly, those additional factors involve an inherent propensity of menstrual tissue to invade and evade capture, ideas which both reflect and reproduce our overall understanding of menstruation as an inherently elusive process.

I want to suggest that in the same sense that references to the disease as 'enigma' work as a metonym for women and femininity, references to menstrual blood and tissue as inherently conniving, evasive, slippery, dynamic and disordered represent a *synecdoche* for women and the feminine. A synecdoche is a rhetorical or literary device where a reference to the part serves as a signifier for the whole. So, for example, an advertisement in which a company announces that it is in need of another 'pair of hands' is a synecdoche, because the part (hands) denotes the whole (person). In the current case, references to menstruation, menstrual blood and tissue functions as a reference to women and the feminine as a whole, where menstrual blood/tissue is understood to be a *component* of femininity. These links are also established via medicine's tendency to conflate retrograde flow with menstruation and women, drawing upon and reiterating the symbolically enigmatic feminine that I discussed earlier. Like the feminine, menstrual blood is slippery, difficult and evasive. The underlying mechanisms of the disease are likely to be associated with the unique attributes and special abilities of menstrual blood and tissue. In this way, yet again, medical literature produces and reproduces a set of important symbolic associations between women, femininity and connivance, performing the disease mechanisms as inherently capable of evading capture. This operates to explain any perceived tensions and inconsistencies *within* theories – such as the retrograde hypothesis – as a function, once again, of the disease's subjects.

Endometriosis is not a Disease at all

The third way that medicine handles the uncertainties, differences and tensions within and between medical theories is to raise questions that are compatible with social constructionist approaches to biomedicine. In 1994, Johannes Evers published a paper in *Human Reproduction* titled 'Endometriosis does not exist; all women have endometriosis'. In that paper, Evers explained:

> These were the provocative conclusions of an endometriosis session held during ESHRE's 7th Annual Meeting, in 1991 in Paris (Evers, 1991). They reflect the opinion that endometrial explants in the peritoneal cavity are a physiological finding in all menstruating women and that, as such, they do not constitute a disease in its proper sense. (1994: 2206)

More recently, Evers (2010: xvii) has revisited this idea, claiming that the title of his 1994 paper was designed:

> To stress that, apart from the many visible lesions, on purely theoretical grounds many more (as yet) invisible lesions can be expected to exist, waiting to develop into visible endometriosis. So it depends on the definition you use and the meticulousness with which you scrutinize the peritoneal cavity whether endometriosis occurs, frequently, always, or not at all.

To understand these ideas more fully, it is worth deviating – very briefly – into the realm of medical history and technology. As with many diseases, the history of endometriosis medicine is one in which surgical techniques and other technological developments are understood to have played a fundamental role in the construction of the disease. As Sarah Evans (2005: 33) explained:

> During the 1980s and 1990s, gynaecologists started taking small samples of tissue called *biopsies* whenever they saw something unusual through the laparoscope. These biopsies were sent to a pathologist for diagnosis using a microscope. By the mid-1990s it became clear that many of these abnormalities were actually endometriosis. Endometriosis became a condition with variable appearance. The lesions could be clear, pink, red or white, as well as black or brown. Once these more subtle lesions were included, it became obvious that endometriosis was a lot more common than once thought. (emphasis in original)

Donnez, Nisolle and Casanas-Roux (1994) argue that these changes led to an increased diagnosis of endometriosis, from 15 per cent in 1986 to 65 per cent in 1988. They argue that the 'increased diagnosis of endometriosis at laparoscopy can be explained by the increased experience and ability of the surgeon to detect such subtle lesions' (Donnez, Nisolle and Casanas-Roux 1994: 342).[3] This demonstrates the fluid nature of disease definitions, as well as the way in which disease boundaries can be mutated via technological interventions and disease

---

3   This was a point also made by Chalmers (1975: 3) who suggested that the apparent increased incidence of endometriosis might have partly been attributable to the more frequent use of laparotomy in recent times.

theory. In recent years the notion of what endometriosis is has evolved to the point where some have claimed it can even be 'invisible'. As Redwine (2003: 65) explains, debates about the possible visual manifestations of endometriosis have been underway since approximately 1985. One controversial form of endometriosis has been discussed in some of the clinical literature. Known as 'invisible microscopic endometriosis' or IME, this is a form of endometriosis which is apparently too small to be detectible during surgery (Redwine 2003: 64). Surgeons who suspect IME might remove a portion of the peritoneum for laboratory testing and if structural changes can be detected in the tissue, the patient is considered to have IME. Different surgeons will thus 'see' things differently (Redwine 2003: 65) and diagnosis may or may not result. For these reasons, Redwine (2003: 67) argues that the 'concept of IME invites scientific and intellectual abuse. If something allegedly exists, but can never be seen, then it can be blamed for anything'. Despite his concerns, Redwine resolves these tensions by valorising the combined capacities of the physician, pathologist and laparoscope to detect endometriosis. He describes the 'identification of endometriosis at surgery [as] an acquired art' (Redwine 2003: 65). Here is yet another instance, then, of the disease's inherent capacity to evade and to confound. As well as reinforcing the overall positioning of the disease as slippery and puzzling, Redwine's account produces medicine as ultimately heroic and omnipotent in the face of the disease, especially where physicians can detect pathology through their 'experience and ability'.

These developments appear to be at the heart of Evers' radically different approach to tensions within the field. Moving between a criticism of the tendency within medicine to identify microscopic and/or 'invisible' lesions, and a celebration of medical precision, Evers' account is open to interpretation. I want to explore at least two possibilities and consider the significance of each. The first possibility is that medicine's problem is one of *definition*, so that tissue found deposited outside the uterus is in fact a normal phenomenon amongst all women. It may represent a precursor to later disease, as some other factors intervene to transform the implant (or explant, in Evers' terms) into an endometrial lesion. Or it may not. Importantly, Evers makes the concession that endometrial explants *are* a form of 'disorder' – although not necessarily a 'disease'. This raises the possibility that retrograde menstruation and implantation is statistically normal, and an inherent form of sickness. Unfortunately, this represents a fairly obvious parallel with historic depictions of women and menstruation in gynaecology. Traditionally, for instance, gynaecology textbooks dismissed complaints related to menstruation, suggesting that women complaining of pain and other symptoms were unlikely to be suffering from any physiological problem, and asserting that no follow-up investigations or treatment were warranted (e.g. Bland-Sutton and Giles 1916; Hermann 1899; Churchill 1885; Atthill 1883). In a comment typical of the discourses around the turn of the twentieth century, Hermann wrote:

> A sensitive patient feels acutely what a strong one would hardly notice. Such a patient may suffer much from the menstrual congestion, although there is *nothing abnormal* except her sensitiveness. Nothing will cure such menstrual pain. (1899: 520, emphasis mine)

Several medical texts claim to have observed a typical psychic demeanour/ personality profile in women who attend clinics complaining of pelvic pain at the menstrual cycle or during sexual intercourse. Hermann argues that spasmodic dysmenorrhoea:

> Occurs in sensitive women. The subjects of it are often tall, well-nourished, not anaemic, intelligent, but always sensitive and often weak … Sometimes we meet with it in undersized, thin, weak, pale patients, who are subject to headache and backache, and cannot bear any strain, mental or physical; in such patients cure is unlikely. (1899: 539)

Atthill was of the view that women who claim to experience menstrual pain were either 'delicate girls of feeble condition', women who lead an inactive life, sempstresses *[sic]*, or overworked servants (1883: 52). Moreover, dysmenorrhoea often developed in women who, although married, had come to regard marriage as a 'positive evil; producing congestion in a malformed organ, and giving rise in turn to a train of distressing symptoms' (Atthill 1883: 61). Churchill considered dysmenorrhoea to be 'almost confined to those [women] of a nervous temperament' (1885: 87). Complaints of pelvic pain were said to be closely associated with a woman's marital status and/or history of childbearing. Unmarried women were said to be more prone to such complaints as well as women (whether married or unmarried) who had not borne children (Churchill 1885: 87; Atthill 1883: 61). The doctor's role was to reassure the woman that her pain was either trivial or imagined (or both):

> The minor gynaecological ailments, real or supposed, are common, and the majority of them come first to the family doctor. He *[sic]* can by sound advice prevent the patient from magnifying trifles; can disabuse her of erroneous theories before they have become fixed in her mind; can dispel her fears for the future; can correct her unhealthy mode of life before it has had time to do harm. (Hermann 1899: 5–6)

The notion that women had 'erroneous' views about pain, views from which she must be disabused were often made on the basis of the author's own clinical observations and anecdotes from practice, extrapolated into unifying statements of 'fact' about the nature and temperament of women. In a similar sense, Evers' claims draw upon and reinforce the possibility that all women are prone to disorder (or that they are always already disordered by virtue of always experiencing menstrual reflux and implantation) and/or that there is no disease at all.

The other possible interpretation is that endometrial tissue found outside the uterus is not indicative of a disease at all, but something experienced by all women. To the extent that symptoms (such as pain) are experienced by some patients, we need to consider other possible sources of that pain. This might accord with the fact that the presence, volume and location of endometrial tissue does not always correspond with the patient's account of symptoms, so that women with little or no endometrial tissue can report acute uterine pain, while women with extensive extra-uterine tissue may report no symptoms at all. Both interpretations create problems for sufferers of endometriosis. If the disease is indeed an all or nothing proposition, then women invariably lose. If all women have endometriosis, and endometriosis is a disease, then all women are diseased. Alternatively, if all women have endometrial explants, and these are merely a 'disorder', but not a 'disease', then all women are disordered. To be sure, medicine is assigned some responsibility for this impossible dilemma, but largely escapes criticism. The problem may even be an effect of medicine's overly 'meticulous' scrutinisation of the pelvis, if not the 'artistry' of its physicians. Somewhat paradoxically, then, even when medicine looks as if it is criticising itself, it continues to perform a trope of science as forever progressive and triumphant. In all of these ways, Evers' 'provocative conclusions' inevitably enact women as the problem – extending a common theme in the medical literature.

Endometriosis is a Set of Diseases

The final example I want to consider involves the propensity within medicine to characterise endometriosis as a collection of diseases. In producing endometriosis as a set of diseases, different theories or aspects of theories that may otherwise be in conflict suddenly emerge with possible validity across an emergent *disease spectrum*. Importantly, endometriosis has not always been understood as a unique or distinctive disease entity (Batt 2011). Despite endometriosis being described as a menstrual disorder, for example, there have been several cases in the medical literature that trouble these characterisations. There have, for instance, been accounts of menstruation appearing in post-menopausal women, or being found outside the pelvis. Endometriosis has been located in the forearm, thigh, small and large intestine and appendix in some cases (Meigs 1953: 47). Similarly, endometriosis has been found in the lung, knee and brain, as I have already mentioned. Crucially, and as I flagged in the Introduction, endometriosis has also been diagnosed in men, raising questions about disease assumptions and classifications that bear in very fundamental ways on our understanding of endometriosis as both a female-specific and gynaecological disease.

Medical literature appears to be responding to these developments by developing *composite* diseases of the kind identified by Annemarie Mol (2002) in her work on atherosclerosis. This is another key strategy for reconciling difference and performing singularity. This strategy is characterised by medicine's production of different disease objects, as in the earlier example of 'walking-atherosclerosis' and 'pressure-atherosclerosis'. Just as it is possible for a patient to have both 'forms' of atherosclerosis at once, it is possible that different patients may express different 'types' of the disease. So, for example, it is increasingly common to see commentators suggest that there are probably several specific *types* of endometriosis, including 'deep infilitrating' endometriosis (Wang, Tokushige, Markham, et al. 2009), 'peritoneal endometriosis' and 'ovarian endometriosis' (Nap 2012).[4] Staying with this trend, Nezhat, Nezhat and Nezhat (2012: 57) recently concluded that endometriosis was probably best understood as 'one name, many diseases'. They argued that what we think of as endometriosis might need to be reimagined in the plural:

> Considering the extraordinary range of morphologies and endlessly disparate reactions endometriosis expresses in response to both surgical and medical interventions, perhaps we are asking the wrong questions. Just as we define cancers today in the plural, we may soon come to recognize endometriosis in the same way: a disorder with multiple phenotypes that share similar molecular mechanisms and reside on that same spectrum, but which manifest differently in each individual as a result of unique ... triggers. (2012: 57–8)

This understanding of the disease positions endometriosis – or perhaps, I should say, *endometrioses* – as less a set of options, as I argued at the start of this chapter, then a set of diseases. As I noted earlier, composite diseases work to *open up* medicine, by introducing the possibility that multiple hypotheses have some relevance to the 'range of morphologies' and 'multiple phenotypes' on display.

There is now explicit recognition of this possibility. Medical literature is increasingly characterised by claims that theories about the diseases are fundamentally interconnected and overlapping. In a recent example of this, Kumar, Tiwari, Sharma, et al. (2012) argue that:

> Several theories have been proposed to explain the pathogenesis of endometriosis – coelomic metaplastic, embryologic and migratory theories. No single theory can account for the location of the ectopic endometrium in all cases of endometriosis.

---

4 Importantly, however, some of the most striking examples of 'difference' (where endometriosis has been identified in men, knees and the brain) tend to be neglected in these processes. The location of the disease in men, for instance, has not led to a wholesale reappraisal of existing knowledge, research and practice, or to a revision of the most basic claims about the disease (that it is a gynaecological condition). Instead, these examples are often described as either simple 'anomalies' or outliers that require a reconsideration of the utility of certain theories (as a challenge, for example, to the retrograde hypothesis).

This burgeoning approach to the disease allows a more sympathetic view of medicine and excludes the need for medicine to produce or select only one theory to explain the disease. So, as Signorile and Baldi (2010: 780) suggested, it is now:

> Possible to claim that endometriosis is a multi-factorial disease with multifaceted features; therefore, all the theories on its pathogenesis must be taken [as] complementary to one another and by no way are mutually exclusive.

Importantly, composite and/or multi-factorial diseases are constituted as components – or perhaps more precisely, *dimensions* – of the same disease object (as opposed to fragmentations). Although multiplicity is acknowledged, overall singularity is preserved. These distributions work to explain away the preponderance of theories, as well as any need to choose between them, rendering the disease as singular, insofar as it is distinct from other diseases – as well as multiple, as a set of interrelated diseases. Importantly, endometriosis is not fragmented into a potentially infinite number of disease states through this process, however, because the number of types is ultimately limited. In this way, medicine contains itself, and its object, and emerges as the 'obligatory point of passage' through which a new range of assessments about the condition should be made. Rather than emerging as fractured, discredited, or incoherent, then, endometriosis disease theories preserve a version of medicine as always, already omnipotent.

Conclusion

In *Aircraft Stories*, Law (2002: 152) suggests that the analysis he undertakes with regards to decision-making:

> Is all very straightforward. Indeed it is obvious to the point of banality. The problem is that its very banality tends to deaden our critical faculties.

The mere articulation of theories about diseases and the decisions that are made about them might also be understood as similarly 'obvious' or 'banal'. Very often, theories are understood to be inert and passive, bearing little relation to 'reality' or 'materiality' beyond the sense in which they purport to represent, interpret, or make sense of that reality. Of course, there *are* instances where theories are understood as having remarkable qualities and important consequences. Take, for example, Einstein's theory of relativity, or Darwin's theory of evolution. Each of these propositions has had a profound effect on the way we understand ourselves and our place in the world. Like many theories from an array of fields, theories such as these represent an exploration of 'big' ideas: about what is possible, probable and likely, as well as who we are, where we have come from and where we may be going. Crucially, however, such theories are often understood as having little utility or import in and of themselves; it is only once they have been interpreted, tested, debated, adapted, developed, challenged, refined, and finally – *fatefully* – taken up, that they will have some impact in and on the world. Even then, most 'ordinary' theories – like the ones I have considered here – will probably be understood as very different to the 'epic' theories or 'grand' narratives articulated by thinkers like Einstein and Darwin. So that while those theories might change the world in some way, other, more 'banal' theories will rarely have *such* an impact.

In this chapter I have argued for a different approach, one in which disease theory is approached as a thoroughly political phenomenon. The significance of medical theory in the present instance emerges partly from the fact that the corpus of endometriosis knowledge and practice is dominated by considerable uncertainty, non-coherence, tension, inconsistency and debate, so that theorisation takes on an even more vital function. In this chapter I have argued that endometriosis is performed as simultaneously multiple and singular, and that various practices of 'holding together' and rationalisation can be identified. What I want to suggest is that more than anything medicine functions to hold *itself* together – as a rational, scientific, heroic, progressive and inherently unified enterprise – even when the proliferation of disease theories might imply inherent chaos, disorder, non-coherence and a lack of order within the field of gynaecological medicine more broadly. As such, uncertainty, non-coherence, tension, inconsistency and debate are actually productive, symbolically and materially. Medicine emerges from the mess and complexity that is understood to be inherent to the disease as unscathed, as well as the counterpoint to the inherently enigmatic feminine. In this way, then, we can conclude that endometriosis theories do two, very important things. First, they perform medicine as heroic and omnipotent, and secondly, they produce/reproduce women as the enigmatic, fundamentally diseased and disordered subjects – indeed, the *necessary objects* – of medical appraisal and intervention. To speak, then, of endometriosis as the 'disease of theories', as Chandler (2000) does, is to speak of a thoroughly politicised set of processes for acting upon the world, enacting gender and distributing agency and power.

Chapter 3

Standing up to the Beast:
On Mystery and Mastery in the
Endometriosis Self-help Literature

Let's look this beast endo straight in the eyes and stand up to it!
(Ballweg and the Endometriosis Association 2003c: 306)

Endometriosis does not control you, you control it.
(Lyons and Kimball 2003: 10)

Self-help literature is one of the central resources that women draw upon during their experiences with endometriosis. Amongst the interviewees for this study, all but three women read self-help literature. Endometriosis self-help books have been the subject of praise in the past, from both academics and health advocates. Ella Shohat (1998: 259), for instance, commended the literature published by the American Endometriosis Association, describing their work as 'feminist' in orientation. The literature comes in for high praise from its readership, as well. Among the women I interviewed for this study, self-help literature was regularly described as of considerable importance and as a source of great comfort. Some of the women I interviewed saw it as offering hope – hope that they might become more empowered in their relations with members of the medical profession and that it may enable them to overcome their physical suffering. As one interviewee, Debbie explained:

> Self-help books as a whole, I guess, apart from just the endo ones, the thing about self-help books, they basically give you your own power back. And that's the thing about reading about endo as well, that I take back control and that I can find answers to my own questions.

In this account, Debbie invokes two common assumptions about endometriosis self-help literature with which I want to engage in this chapter. The first is the notion that self-help books *act upon the subject in certain ways*: either by creating or heightening a capacity within them to act upon the world. In this sense, Debbie's account raises questions about the relationship between self-help literature and agency. The second idea rendered visible in Debbie's account is that self-help literature has an inherently informative function: illuminating, perhaps, complex medical issues or areas of uncertainty. In so doing, self-help books provide 'answers' to the many questions that women may have – whether they are about causation, diagnosis, treatment or prognosis. This idea – that self-help books may assist women to reach a better understanding of what endometriosis is and how to treat it – was regularly articulated in the interviews I conducted for this research. Importantly, then, Debbie articulates two common conceptions about self-help books: that they are transformative in their potential and informative in their content. Academics have given much consideration to claims about both the transformative potential and informative nature of self-help books. Despite the apparent centrality of endometriosis literature to women's experiences, and the potential socio-cultural significance of self-help literature in health more broadly, however, no study that I am aware of has examined the content of endometriosis self-help literature. This chapter involves a critical examination of 11 full-length self-help books dedicated to endometriosis, along with two chapters from more general books on women's health.[1]

In what follows, I argue that in spite of various medical and scientific uncertainties about endometriosis, self-help literature enacts endometriosis as a largely stable and 'knowable' object. Alongside this, self-help books produce women as intrinsically capable of managing and even preventing the disease. In short, then, self-help books eschew medical configurations of the disease as principally enigmatic and *mysterious*, producing endometriosis as capable of being *mastered*. The way agency is materialised in self-help books is fundamental to these configurations, with the literature underpinned by a very particular kind of subject/object relation. This subject/object relation, I suggest, is an essential component in the discursive power of self-help books, to the extent such power exists. Interestingly, self-help books produce and reproduce a version of women's agency that looks, on the face of it, to be at odds with traditional understandings of women's agency. Constituted as potentially masterful, self-help books enact women in ways that seem to challenge to orthodox understandings and representations of them as 'passive', weak, irrational and sick. I critically

---

1   I found 11 full-length self-help books for women with endometriosis suitable for study. These are *Endometriosis* by Julia Older (1984), *Coping with Endometriosis* by Jo Mears (1996), *Explaining Endometriosis* by Lorraine Henderson and Ros Wood (2000), *Coping with Endometriosis* by Robert Phillips and Glenda Motta (2000), *Endometriosis: A Key to Healing through Nutrition* (2002) by Mills and Vernon, *What to Do When the Doctor Says it's Endometriosis* (2003) by Lyons and Kimball, *Endometriosis: The Complete Reference for Taking Charge of your Health* (2003) by Ballweg and the Endometriosis Association, *Endometriosis and Other Pelvic Pain* (2005) by Evans, *Endometriosis for Dummies* (2007) by Krotec and Perkins, *Take Control of Your Endometriosis: Help Relieve Symptoms with Simple Diet and Lifestyle Changes* by Henrietta Norton (2012), and *Reclaim Your Life: Your Guide to Aid Healing of Endometriosis* by Carolyn Levett (2008). The chapters examined in full-length women's health and/or gynaecology books were: 'Soothing the Hurt: Endometriosis and Pelvic Pain' in *Healing Mind, Healthy Woman* (1996) by Alice Domar and Henry Dreher and 'Endometriosis' in *Women's Bodies, Women's Wisdom* (1998) by Dr Christiane Northrup. A more detailed explanation of the methods used to analyse the texts appears in Seear (2009a).

evaluate these claims, however, focussing on the ways in which self-help books materialise a version of agency that is ultimately more *consistent* with traditional understandings of women and femininity than *antithetical* to them. The political, ethical and material dimensions of these enactments are considered, especially insofar as they re/produce 'responsibilised' subjects, with implications for medicine, epidemiology and public health.

How Texts Relate to the World

As I explained in the Introduction, John Law (2002) argues for a very particular understanding of the importance of texts and the way that texts 'relate to the world'. So, it will be recalled, Law argues that texts do not merely *represent* reality – they participate in the *making* of reality (or, more precisely, realities). Law's observations bear directly on the question of how we should study texts. What questions should we ask about them, given the shift in emphasis (and the action of the text) signaled by Law? The French philosopher Gilles Deleuze famously made the point that the framing of questions not only informs the answers one gets, but enacts the reality or 'truth' pertaining to the problem in question:

> A solution always has the truth it deserves according to the problem to which it is a response, and the problem always has the solution it deserves in proportion to its own truth or falsity – in other words, in proportion to its sense. (Deleuze, 1994: 158)

Following this approach, and as I have argued in my previous work with Suzanne Fraser (Fraser and Seear 2011: 46):

> The kinds of questions we posit about an area of inquiry can themselves be revealing. If we ask, for instance, whether a thing is represented "accurately", we assume, and, in so doing, enact, a single perspective on reality (this much is implied by the form of the inquiry itself – that there is a stable reality that can be represented "accurately").[2]

As we argued in our work on hepatitis C, these ideas force us to ask certain kinds of questions. Although there are many questions that one could ask, such as what self-help books do with biomedicine, biomedical treatment, alternative treatment,

---

2   This approach can be contrasted to several extant studies of self-help literature which have instead explored questions associated with the psychometric and rational-actor models of risk analysis. These studies have focussed on the extent to which self-help literature actually 'amplifies' risks (see Kasperson, Renn, Slovic, et al. 1988 for more), thus depending upon and reproducing a realist understanding of risk.

and the like, I confine myself to just two questions in this chapter. Rather than asking: 'How do self-help books represent endometriosis?', or perhaps even 'Do self-help books accurately represent endometriosis and endometriosis medicine?', it is more useful to ask: 'What do self-help books do with endometriosis?', and also 'What do self-help books do with the endometriotic subject?' These are the main two questions that I explore in this chapter. By extension, I also consider how self-help books deal with the relationship between disease and subject.

Before embarking upon my analysis, it is important to make the point, as with my previous work (e.g. Fraser and Seear 2011) that reality is multiple (Mol 2002). What this means is that that the version (or versions) of endometriosis that materialise in self-help books may differ in important ways from the versions that appear elsewhere, such as in medical literature or clinical practice. To the extent, moreover, that self-help books enact the disease, and to the extent that self-help books are not always uniform in their approach, it is possible that there is more than one version of endometriosis materialised in the self-help literature. As I explained in the introductory chapter, however, the notion that reality is multiple must be distinguished from the notion that it is plural, so that although, following Mol (2002), there may be 'more than one' version of endometriosis, there is still 'less than many'. The process of exploring the enactment of endometriosis in self-help books is therefore complicated by variances within and between books, as well as variations that may emerge over time, as medical theories, treatments and practices change.

My analysis is further complicated by at least two more factors, each of which is flagged by both Law and Deleuze. I recognise that the approach I take in this chapter works to enact a version (or versions) of the disease, and that this has its own political and ethical implications. In addition, of course, the way endometriosis is performed herein may differ from the way it might be performed elsewhere, especially insofar as others studying the disease might want to ask different questions. This leads me to the question of interpretation in academic analysis, because as well as the fact that I might ask a different set of questions than someone else, I may also interpret the literature differently. My interpretations may be shaped by a range of things including, of course, my own experiences with the disease. In this respect, the comments I made in the introduction to this book on writing remain relevant. The account I offer in this chapter, then, neither purports to be the only way self-help books might be read, nor to be a definitive analysis of the way these books function. Mine is necessarily a partial account of how endometriosis self-help books may operate. Despite all of this, I consider this to be a valuable and hopefully provocative analysis that seeks to encourage debate about self-help books and how they approach disease. I say this in part because, as I flagged at the start of this chapter, endometriosis self-help literature has been met enthusiastically in most circles (including academia). As I will argue in what follows, that enthusiasm, well perhaps well-founded in some respects, might also need to be tempered with some concern.

Historical Perspectives on Self-help Literature

Self-help literature is not a new phenomenon. It first emerged in the seventeenth century in the form of religious self-help literature (Starker 1989) and proliferated throughout the nineteenth century (Grodin 1991). Production and distribution increased steadily after the late 1930s (Simonds 1992), exploding in popularity after the 1970s (Ehrenreich and English 1978).[3] Simonds suggests that the genre has 'gradually gained a significant place within the trade and mass-market book publishing industries in the United States' (1992: 3). Individuals are increasingly turning to self-help literature for solutions to a whole range of life's problems, with most readers of self-help literature being women (Simonds 1996, 1992; Starker 1986).[4] This raises the question of why is there an increasing interest in self-help books. Hochschild (1994) suggests that it may be a consequence of a decreasing emphasis on traditional forms of authority such as the church and family in late modernity. Simonds (1992: 5), on the other hand, suggests that the popularity of self-help literature (within America at least) may be the result of an increasing self-interest among individuals. The preoccupation with the self as a project has been identified as a defining characteristic of late modernity (Giddens 1991). These are all possibilities, of course, but I argue that the relationship between self-help books, the decreasing emphasis on traditional forms of authority and the self as a project is much more likely to be more fluid and dynamic than this: a mutually constitutive process, shaped by the processes of reading and interpretation, as well as the specific and local arrangement of subjects, objects and subject matter within self-help books.

Perhaps the first book to directly speak to women about endometriosis was the publication *Our bodies, ourselves* produced by The Boston Women's Health Book Collective (BWHBC) in 1973. The book was a comprehensive manual written for women, by women, about women's bodies and was aimed at empowering 'lay' women in their encounters with the medical profession. Endometriosis received brief attention in the first edition of the book (BWHBC 1973: 261), warranting four short paragraphs. This was enough only for a very brief description of the disease and its principal symptoms. By 1984, the BWHBC's new edition of the early self-help book contained a much more detailed analysis of the condition. Stretching over approximately two and a half pages, the authors comprehensively criticised the 'career women's' label described elsewhere in this book, as well as highlighting traditional, 'anachronistic' views about the disease (BWHBC 1984: 501). These

---

3   For a very detailed explanation of the social and cultural context within which self-help literature became popular amongst mainstream Americans throughout the twentieth century, see Starker (1989).

4   However books written specifically for men are becoming increasingly common (Singleton 2004, 2003).

books signalled the start of a more formal lay discourse about endometriosis and in 1984, the first full-length endometriosis self-help book appeared (Older 1984).[5]

The endometriosis self-help literature, at least in part, had its origins in the ideology of the women's health movement, which aimed to challenge how medical knowledge was applied to women. One of the stated aims of early self-help literature addressing endometriosis was to empower women patients to challenge anachronistic thinking regarding menstrual pain and the 'proper' role of women and to become informed, responsible, self-reliant and capable agents in their own care. Although endometriosis self-help literature may have its origins in a feminist philosophy concerned with challenging medical power-knowledge and the status quo and while it may in part operate as such, I argue that the texts also function to produce and reproduce the status quo. That is, endometriosis self-help literature renders women subjects as responsible for disease causation, risk management and prevention – an arrangement that differs little from many earlier 'anachronistic' representations of which self-help authors are universally critical. Self-help books produce and reproduce a highly individualised health ethic which is closely aligned with a neoliberal perspective on the subject's role in health care. Also, as I will argue in this chapter, self-help authors construct the self as ontologically separate from – and superior to – the body and as capable of mastering several dimensions of illness. I raise a series of concerns about this configuration. One cause for concern lies in the very notion that disease can be controlled. Is it possible, realistic or likely that women with endometriosis can successfully manage their disease, prevent disease recurrence or progression, overcome their pain or infertility through action? If so, what kind of action is needed in order to achieve this, and what resources is such action premised upon? What is the likelihood that women will have access to such resources and what are some of the implications where access is not possible? In this chapter I explore these issues and highlight concerns around the notion, present in many

---

5   This raises the question: what is a self-help book? Identifying self-help books is no easy task, especially as there are no established criteria for what constitutes a self-help book (Starker 1989: 8) and self-help literature is a fluid concept. As Simonds (1992: 3) found, readers of self-help literature often describe the genre in a very diverse way. In order that this study be manageable, it was important that to set some parameters in order to narrow down the field of potential texts for study. As such, I considered that endometriosis self-help literature could be defined as any text purporting to contain detailed advice about this condition of both an informative and therapeutic nature and directed towards a lay audience. I consider these to be the common qualities of self-help literature (although the definition of 'endometriosis self-help literature' is by no means closed, and I recognise that my selection of books also works to perform the 'genre' of self-help literature in a very specific way). I sought to examine endometriosis self-help literature that traversed a broad range of subjects (for example: medical treatments, alternative therapies, emotional and lifestyle issues) and that might broadly fall within the recognised attributes of the self-help genre (it was directed at a lay audience and had an informative and/or therapeutic intent of some kind).

self-help books, that endometriosis is simultaneously a disease of 'risk' but that risks can be avoided or even 'controlled'. On the one hand, this is a potentially paradoxical claim. On the other, give the range of apparent risk variables that circulate in self-help literature, it seems unlikely, if not impossible, that women could successfully avoid all risks. In what follows I highlight several other tensions and concerns in the literature, especially around the way self-help books 'handle' gender, femininity and the agency of women. I argue that the content of the endometriosis self-help literature generates a series of major political and ethical problems, and conclude with a few suggestions about how these books might be revised in future.

Enacting the Disease

The first and perhaps most obvious observation that can be made about endometriosis self-help literature is that it – like the other texts I have discussed in this book to date – enacts the disease. As we know, medical literature on endometriosis is usually characterised by a focus on one or more discrete issues: the biological 'features', for instance, of the disease, treatment regimens and efficacy, or the likely disease mechanisms. In contrast, endometriosis self-help literature tends to adopt a much wider focus, and by extension, to enact the disease as a complex and multi-faceted phenomenon comprised of various emotional and psychological dimensions.[6] Endometriosis is typically described as a chronic illness, which, although understood as a gynaecological disease, effects women in ways that extend far beyond the 'merely' physical. Take, for example, the opening pages of Lyons and Kimball's (2003: 9–10) book *What to Do When the Doctor Says it's Endometriosis*, which opens with the question 'What is endometriosis?' In this passage, the emphasis is upon the chronic and disabling nature of the disease for many women:

> For women with endometriosis, the answer to "what is it?" is simple: Endometriosis is what's keeping you from living your life to the fullest. Because endometriosis causes pain, as well as other symptoms, this problem keeps some women in bed for several days each month. Other women have chronic low-level pain that just hangs on day after day after day with little relief. And some have menstrual flow so heavy that they can't stray too far from a bathroom and a supply of feminine products. You can't plan a weekend away because you just

---

6 Almost all texts dedicate sections (or chapters) to the emotional effects of having a chronic illness, including a consideration of the impact of endometriosis on a woman's sexual and personal relationships (although a heterosexual orientation is assumed), working life and fertility. Most texts conclude with a chapter about the future: how to live with a chronic illness, how to take control of your life and health care regime, or how to develop an effective support network of friends, family and medical staff.

don't know if you will be up for the trip. Since your teenage years, you were the family "sick kid". No reunion, family picnic, or holiday gathering went by without you either feeling too ill to attend or curled up in your aunt's bedroom unable to participate in the fun. Endometriosis impacts a woman's ability to develop a relationship or to maintain an intimate relationship. Sex is often painful. And to top it off, endometriosis often compromises fertility, making it difficult to conceive.

In *Endometriosis for Dummies* (2007: 1), Krotec and Perkins explain that endometriosis is 'a chronic disease' with various symptoms that until recently were understood 'as being more psychological than physical in origin'. Explaining the potentially widespread range of symptoms women may experience and the personal and social impacts of the disease, the authors explain that:

> Endometriosis is far more than just cramps. Millions of dollars are lost in the workplace each year because of absences and surgeries related to endometriosis. Endometriosis symptoms can cause everything from headaches to chest pain – in addition to the more common symptoms of cramps, painful sex, and abnormal bleeding. Many women with endometriosis have suffered for years without realizing that they had a serious disease (and may have been called *malingerers*, fakers who use illness to avoid work) because their disease wasn't visible! Too often these women have given up on getting help. (2007: 1; emphasis in original)

Usually, descriptions such as these are accompanied by assertions about the ways women living with endometriosis will *feel* about their illness. It is typically suggested that women diagnosed with endometriosis will express emotions including helplessness, hopelessness, depression, anxiety, fear, anger, resentment, isolation and bitterness. Assertions such as these might resonate with sufferers, especially as most women living with endometriosis report having had their symptoms and feelings dismissed by the medical profession (Henderson and Wood 2000: 137). Regardless of how individual women respond to these characterisations, endometriosis self-help literature constitutes endometriosis 'holistically' – as more than a 'merely' biomedical phenomenon or physical disease state. Self-help books therefore tend to materialise endometriosis, variously, as a chronic, incurable, or disabling condition, with a range of possibly devastating personal, emotional and financial 'effects'. To the extent that endometriosis is constituted as wide-ranging in its effects, as we shall see, it also figures as a disease that demands comprehensive attention.

As a disease with seemingly wide-ranging implications, endometriosis self-help literature offers apparently comprehensive information about all 'aspects' of the disease. In *Coping with Endometriosis*, for example, it is said that:

> Experts just don't have all the answers, and this can be frustrating and upsetting. Even worse is the feeling of isolation you may experience, the feeling that you're

all alone because no one understands. This can be really depressing ... But that's why this book was written. It is chock-full of information, suggestions, and strategies to help you, your doctor, your family, and your friends learn how to successfully cope with endometriosis. (Phillips and Motta 2000: xi)

In this excerpt, a sharp distinction is drawn between the solutions made available via mainstream medicine and those that women will find in self-help. Here, Phillips and Motta seem to be suggesting that although 'experts' don't have all of the answers, self-help authors might. At the very least, it is implied that self-help books can offer more to women than other 'experts'. This passage also flags the apparently central role of the endometriotic subject in self-help literature. Phillips and Motta claim that their role is to 'help' women 'learn how to successfully cope' with the disease. This implies that women are at the centre of the book – rather than periphery – and that the authors' task is to help enable women to build their capacities in a project of learning and coping. This indicates a particular kind of subject-object configuration within self-help literature that I will come back to.

As well as constituting endometriosis as a disease with wide-ranging 'effects', self-help books adopt an ambivalent and at times contradictory approach to what the disease 'is'. As I argued in the previous chapter, medical literature performs endometriosis as enigmatic and mysterious, emphasising theoretical pluralism and the central role of science in seeking to understand the disease. Self-help books reiterate aspects of this, highlighting the extant medical uncertainties about the disease's origins, mechanisms and treatment options, the apparent spike in disease incidence and prevalence and the changing nature of the disease. In this sense, self-help books play a part in producing and reproducing endometriosis as a 'crisis of the modern'. The disease is also constituted as difficult to understand and to detect: there may be variations in the appearance of lesions, for example, which come in differing colours, shapes and sizes. Such lesions may even be 'camouflaged' (Norton 2012: 12) as something else. Doubt is also cast upon the role of hormones and whether or not the disease is cyclical in nature. The fact that endometrial tissue can be found outside the uterus is constructed as the source of further confusion. Partly because of this, questions are raised about how the disease should be categorised: is it a gynaecological or immunological condition? In all of these ways, self-help books reflect and reproduce medical understandings of endometriosis as a largely incoherent object. Importantly, however, self-help books also enact their own versions of the disease. This involves – somewhat confusingly – a tendency to enact endometriosis as a largely stable object. Endometriosis is also constructed as a 'simple' (Lyons and Kimball 2003: 9) disease, with specific effects and symptoms (albeit wide-ranging), and as something that can be known, rationalised, coped with, and managed. I am especially interested in this notion – that despite its variability and apparent complexity, endometriosis can be comprehended, contained and even controlled. The subject, as we shall see, is central to this process of rationalisation and containment, a vastly different approach to the disease than the one that emerges through the biomedical literature.

I now turn to questions about the disease-subject relation and the way self-help books constitute agency.

Enacting Agency

The stated aim of many endometriosis self-help books is straightforward: their purpose is to provide women with information about the disease, its possible causes and how it can be treated. In perhaps the first ever self-help book on endometriosis, author Julia Older (1984: xvii) said that the purpose of her book was:

> to present the many viewpoints, the controversial theories and contradictory data, so that women everywhere may at least have access to it.

Self-help authors do not simply seek to increase women's access to information about endometriosis, however. They aim to also motivate them to take action, propagating the idea that women can manage the disease and their symptoms, or even prevent it from recurring or proliferating. The central message of self-help books is that endometriosis can be overcome. The titles of the books I analysed for this chapter are indicative of this approach, with references to women 'healing' (Mills and Vernon 2002), 'coping' (Phillips and Motta 2000), 'taking charge' (Ballweg and the Endometriosis Association 2003), taking 'control' (Norton 2012) and 'reclaiming' (Levett 2008) their lives. In this respect, women are constituted as agentive, by which I mean they are positioned as having the capacity to act upon their disease in a range of ways. What this also means is that one of the central functions of self-help books is that they enact a very particular disease-subject relation, where women figure as superior to endometriosis, because they have the capacity to variously manage, control, avoid or otherwise *act upon* it.

The introduction to Mills and Vernon's (2002) *Endometriosis: A Key to Healing through Nutrition* is perhaps the best example of this approach. That book begins with the following series of assertions around self, body and disease:

> You have a key to good health. Your body wants to be well, that is its natural state. Endometriosis is a jigsaw puzzle of symptoms. You need to fit all the pieces together to provide clues as to what is happening within your body. This book will try to give you some of the pieces of the jigsaw, but you have to put them together yourself. This book will guide you to a truth. As you will read in the following chapters, some pioneering women have taken this path before and they share their success with you. Let them lead the way. They have found that by giving the body the building blocks it needs, health can be regained. That is the key, which you must always remember. Your body wants to be well. (2002: 1)

This is a complex passage in which several of the main tenets of self-help literature can be found. First, a state of full 'health' is produced as inherently normal, 'natural' and desirable. Endometriosis is constituted as an intrinsically 'puzzling' disease, reiterating medical depictions of the disease as enigmatic and mysterious. Crucially, however, the apparent mysteriousness of the disease is something that can be solved. Adopting a vastly different approach to the medical literature, this account, like many others in the self-help literature, performs an ontological separation between a woman's body and self, with the latter having its own independent motivations and 'wants' (namely, 'to be well'). Despite the body having its own capacities and desires, Mills and Vernon construct the self as superior to – and capable of mastering – the body. This mastery is possible through various means, including the accurate interpretation of the body's 'clues', putting together the pieces of the jigsaw puzzle, or, less specifically, accessing the 'truth'.

Similar messages can be found in most other books. Positioning readers as agentive and ultimately capable of acting upon their illness in important ways, women are encouraged to 'not despair. Let's look this beast endo straight in the eyes and stand up to it!' (Ballweg and the Endometriosis Association 2003c: 306). The aim, in short, is to learn how the disease works so that the woman living with endometriosis can 'fight endometriosis and win' (Mills and Vernon 2002: 2). Readers of the self-help literature are encouraged to 'seize the day and develop a whole new attitude' (Lyons and Kimball 2003: 10), and to take action to increase their 'body's chances of coping with and perhaps overcoming [their] endometriosis' (Henderson and Wood 2000, 92–5). Indeed, a central premise of the self-help literature is 'that endometriosis does not control you, *you control it*' (Lyons and Kimball 2003: 10; my emphasis). Women are encouraged to control the disease by 'taking charge' of their bodies and minds. Each woman needs to accept her disease and seek to make change: 'This book was written to help you take charge of your body and to become an active rather than a passive participant in your treatment plan' (Phillips and Motta 2000: xii).

So how is this to be achieved? How, that is, are women to take control of their illness? One of the first steps is for women to uncover the 'reasons' that endometriosis developed:

> If all of us have the potential for endometriosis, why do some women develop symptoms while others do not? Since the medical authorities cannot tell us, the answers lie within the individual woman. It is up to her to decipher what her symptoms are trying to tell her. (Northrup 1998: 165)[7]

---

7 Northrup is of the view that endometriosis often occurs in women who have experienced sexual abuse (1998: 19–20, 41) or stress (1998: 164). In *Healing Mind, Healthy Woman* Domar and Dreher (1996: 367) make a similar point. They write: 'My own clinical experience bears this out – pelvic-pain patients frequently report an abuse history, ongoing abuse in current relationships, extreme stress, and feelings of despair. I find that these patients often respond extremely well to cognitive and behavioral therapies.'

As with the earlier example from Mills and Vernon (2002), this excerpt produces and reproduces a Cartesian distinction between the subject's 'self' and her 'body'. Women are told to 'listen to the messages that their bodies give them' (Mills and Vernon 2003: 232). Although the body is positioned as agentive – it *gives* messages to the self – the literature unequivocally positions the self as having a superior function as regards the body. In the main, the role of the 'self' is to assist the 'body' to overcome illness: 'the body needs help in order to rid itself of the "rogue" tissue of endometriosis' (Mills and Vernon 2003: 3).

In manufacturing an ontological separation of self and body, these books invoke a device commonly utilised in the spiritual and psychological self-help literature, where individuals are constructed as possessing 'an inner reservoir of power that can be accessed' (Rimke 2000: 64). According to Rimke (2000), these constructions are usually accompanied by injunctions to individuals to take some kind of action. In psychological self-help literature, the focus may be on therapy and other practices associated with the 'psy' culture. In health self-help books, the focus may include psychological 'work' along with other activities. Regardless of the specific injunctions involved, the point is that self-help literature often produces a set of expectations that render individuals as responsible for their own health, well-being and so on. Individuals are expected to do something to access their 'inner reservoir of power'. The notion that individuals can harness their 'inner power' bears close resemblance to Nikolas Rose's (1999) idea of autonomous selfhood. According to Rose, the autonomous self is a central feature of late modernity: individuals are understood as capable of autonomous action, and obliged to construct their own biographies. The rhetoric associated with autonomous selfhood suggests that 'we are not what we are, but what we make of ourselves' (Giddens 1991: 68). Rose is critical of these demands, however, suggesting that the 'assertions of autonomy, individuality, selfhood and self-mastery' associated with autonomous selfhood are 'if not illusory, then imaginary' (Rose 1999: xxiv). This is because there is an 'inherent sociality of being' (Rimke 2000: 62) and because all our lives are restrained to some extent by the 'material and cultural framework' (Daykin and Naidoo 1995: 61) within which we live. As we will see, the endometriosis self-help literature largely neglects these dimensions, however, promulgating the notion that 'people can exercise mastery of themselves and their lives' (Rimke 2000: 62). In the next sections I look more closely at what it is that women with endometriosis are being called upon to master; how, in particular, theories of the disease and disease causation materialise in self-help books, and some of the problems associated with this.

Enacting Disease Theories

Many texts offer explanations for women developing the condition. Common reasons include that endometriosis results from psychological dysfunction, or that it is caused by stress or anxious thinking.[8] In *Women's Bodies, Women's Wisdom*, Christiane Northrup argues that the disease is not 'just medical' but instead that it is related to 'other parts of our lives' (1998: 22). From here, she continues:

> Endometriosis is the illness of competition. It comes about when a woman's emotional needs are competing with her functioning in the outside world. When a woman feels that her innermost emotional needs are in direct conflict with what the world is demanding of her, endometriosis is one of the ways in which her body tries to draw her attention to the problem. (Northrup 1998: 163)

Whilst Northrup says it can be harmful for women to fall into the trap of blaming themselves for causing their illnesses, she nevertheless encourages women to look at mind–body connections in a way that has the potential to lead to such a conclusion: 'Our illnesses often exist to get our attention and get us back on track' (Northrup 1998: 43).

Constituting the disease as both a disease and a symptom of the subject's relationship to herself, endometriosis is constructed as the body's way of getting a woman's 'attention' and of 'trying not to let us forget our feminine nature, our need for self-nurturance and our connection with other women' (Northrup 1998).

In this example, the notion of women having a feminine essence surfaces, and is constructed as crucial to the disease's development. Because of this apparently causal connection, women suffering from the disease are enjoined to try and establish a closer connection with this feminine 'nature'. These ideas function to achieve at least three things. First, this passage enacts 'femininity' as both distinct from 'masculinity' and as being made up of, among other things, a need for self-nurturance. Secondly, it produces women as responsible, and responsible for becoming more 'feminine', because being more attentive and connected to femininity is crucial to the management of the disease. Thirdly, because a disordered relationship with one's femininity might trigger gynaecological problems, women are produced as both vulnerable – and close – to nature. In constructing the disease as an expression of disordered femininity, then, Northrup is performing a set of fundamentally gendered ideas about women, nature and health. In a similar sense, the authors of *Healing Mind, Healthy Woman* suggest that 'the mind is at the heart of women's health' (Domar and Dreher 1996: xxiii). Like Northrup, Domar and Dreher (1996) perform endometriosis in ways that are familiar, and aligned with traditional biomedical understandings of the disease

---

8 Specific symptoms of endometriosis are also positioned as resulting from women's psyche. In relation to infertility, for instance, Northrup (1998: 168) writes: 'Endometriosis has been clearly associated with decreased female egg fertilisation, decreased success rates for in vitro fertilisation ("test tube" fertilisation) and increased miscarriages. The clinical experience of therapist Niravi Payne with women with infertility and endometriosis clearly shows that, at an unconscious level, these women may be ambivalent about becoming pregnant. Their minds may desire it, while their hearts aren't sure.'

as psychogenic or psychosomatic. Rather than challenging medical theories or practices that perform endometriosis as a function of women's minds, then, self-help books actually operate to reinforce them. As these examples also show, the endometriosis self-help literature performs gender in ways that are generally compatible with existing stereotypes.

Earlier in this book, I identified a number of medical theories about what causes endometriosis. In the 1970s and '80s, endometriosis was thought to be a 'career women's disease' – a condition occurring amongst women who have pursued careers at the expense of performing the more traditional roles of childbearing and housekeeping. In the endometriosis self-help literature, the 'career woman' label is often explicitly criticised. However in an odd contradiction, the remnants of the 'career woman' hypothesis can still be located in the literature, albeit couched in slightly different language. In *Endometriosis*, for example, Older (1984) includes a section called 'Were you meant to have 425 periods – or 50?' where the author laments the shift away from traditional childbearing roles and suggests that this might cause or contribute to endometriosis. In an extended section early in her text, even before explaining what endometriosis is – Older addresses these concerns in an alarmist way:

> We cannot escape the twentieth century. But we can consider our own priorities in respect to the outside world and in relation to the intimate and innate system of our bodies. Let us hope that women will take the initiative. Even if it is too late for our generation, at least we may begin to explain to our daughters the physiological consequences that sometimes accompany certain life decisions. These are facts that girls should be told, not just at puberty ... but before, when questions arise about menstruation. Item: By the age of thirty-five to thirty-nine years, their chances for pregnancy will have decreased by 20 percent. Item: Endometriosis is the leading cause of infertility in women in their twenties. In approximately 40 to 50 percent of these cases, the infertility will be permanent. Item: Long periods of ovulation without interruption (for whatever reason) can predispose women to endometriosis. If these important considerations are explained to twelve-and thirteen-year olds in tandem with the facts of life, fewer women tomorrow will suffer from pain, the adverse side effects of medical and surgical treatment, and the sometimes irreversible damage to their reproductive systems. Early information and knowledge will help women to recognise endometriosis and will assist them in choosing the direction of their lives without fear. (Older 1984: 9)

In more recent literature, this theme is continued. Where theories about what causes endometriosis are addressed, attention is given to the possibility that women who are 'putting off' (Domar and Dreher 1996: 364) pregnancy or breastfeeding are at a greater risk of developing endometriosis (Henderson and Wood 2000: 12–15, 118–19; Northrup 1998: 165; Mears 1996: 2). Rather than subverting dominant medical discourses, then, some self-help literature reproduces the notion that women's lifestyle choices are the cause of endometriosis. In many cases, medical theory is merely incorporated into the self-help literature – without challenge – with the authors simply amending the medical jargon to make it more accessible. Endometriosis is thus constituted as a disease caused by women's psyche, lifestyle, sexual and reproductive choices. In all of these ways women surface as responsible for managing it. As these examples also show, the function and management of emotions runs through the existing literature. In the next section I consider emotion management in more detail.

Keeping Up Appearances: Agency and Emotions

As the theorist of race and culture Sara Ahmed (2004a, 2004b) has compellingly argued, emotions, like any 'thing', are not anterior to social relations. According to Ahmed, a conventional approach to emotions understands them as something that people hold or own. Emotions emerge from within the subject and are expressed outwardly, towards things (places, objects) as well as to people. We express 'love' towards our friends and family, or 'hate' towards our enemies. We feel 'guilty', experience 'shame', 'anger', 'fear' and 'loathing'. Instead, Ahmed argues, the practice of articulating emotions – rather than simply attaching to existing subjects – actually functions to bring those subjects into being. So, when an individual expresses 'hatred' towards a person of Aboriginal descent, for example, the articulation enacts Aboriginal persons as separate from non-Aboriginals. The same processes can be identified at work in the endometriosis self-help literature, concerned as it is with the place of emotions in the lives of women with endometriosis.

As already noted, women with endometriosis are assumed to experience certain emotions. These feelings may be 'about' the diagnosis, or the symptoms, the effects of the disease on their relationships, work, fertility and sexuality, or emerging out of the way women have been treated by doctors. Importantly, the self-help literature encourages them to contain and control these emotions, primarily because they are a hindrance to a rational and reasoned strategy of managing chronic illness. In *Coping with Endometriosis*, Phillips and Motta (2000: 43) suggest that 'one of the most important aspects of coping with endometriosis is the ability to control your emotions'. Women are encouraged to replace negative emotions with 'more rational, realistic and positive' thoughts (Phillips and Motta 2000: 48), to 'improve' their feelings (Lyons and Kimball 2003: 243) and to manage their emotional responses. Even if a woman does not feel in control of her emotions, she should still present a public face of happiness:

> Keep up your appearance, and try to be cheerful. Believe it or not, the very act of seeming cheerful often leads to feeling this way. So walk tall and hold your head high. Feel good about who you are. (Phillips and Motta 2000: 52)

The need for women to 'keep up appearances' is an extension of the 'imperatives of femininity' (Stacey 1997: 197), whereby women are expected to perform themselves in particular ways and to put the needs of others first, presumably based on the assumption that this will benefit others. What we see here is the enactment of two 'sets' of emotions: those symbolically adjacent to chaos, on the one hand (negativity, irrational and idealistic) and those associated with order, on the other (positivity, rationality and realism, among other things). Importantly, these renderings also belie a symbolic association with yet another crucial binary pair: the 'feminine' (associated with chaos) and the 'masculine' (symbolically linked to order). The endometriosis self-help literature therefore produces and reproduces a set of ideal subjects: the 'proper' rational/masculine/ ordered subject who controls her emotions in the face of her illness and remains 'cheerful' in spite of everything, and the 'disavowed' irrational/feminine/chaotic subject, who fails to (adequately and appropriately) control her emotions.

A number of texts, such as *Explaining Endometriosis* (Henderson and Wood 2000) and *Coping with Endometriosis* (Phillips and Motta 2000) also dedicate a section to discussing how others will feel once a woman has been diagnosed with endometriosis. Special attention is often given to how (male) partners might feel. Women are encouraged to think about others, to recognise that their (male) partners will likely need to talk about their feelings, that they will feel distressed at changes in their sexual relationship and that they will need to feel that they are still loved (Henderson and Wood 2000: 163). In *Coping with Endometriosis*, women are encouraged to avoid 'constantly badgering' their partner and to avoid 'pointing out how things must change because of [their] condition' (Phillips and Motta 2000: 236). Where a partner is having trouble adjusting to changes that result from living with endometriosis, she is advised to 'concentrate on improving [her] own thoughts and feelings', (Phillips and Motta 2000: 236) towards his response. The advice is directed at her, not at him. Her tolerant attitude towards her partner should be the focal point:

> Eileen, a 38-eight-year-old *[sic]* mother of two, told her husband, Alan, that at times he would have to shop for food, prepare the meals, and clean the house – because she was in too much pain. Their two teenage children would have to help out as well. Despite the fact that Eileen's family loved her and was concerned about her health, they were understandably upset. Her husband was especially distressed since he knew little about cooking. How can you make changes as smoothly as possible, without causing your partner unnecessary distress? First, make the changes gradually. Try to avoid overwhelming any family member. And be realistic in your expectations, keeping in mind that it takes time for anyone to comfortably incorporate new responsibilities into their normal routine. (Phillips and Motta 2000: 235–6)

Women are also encouraged to 'discuss changes *reasonably* and *be gentle*' (Phillips and Motta 2000: 236; emphasis added).

Eileen's story is troublesome for several reasons. Most importantly, the story reproduces and endorses traditional gender roles and expectations. Eileen's request for assistance is portrayed as 'a favour' from Alan, presumably because she is responsible for maintaining the effective operation of the home. She has to consult her husband about the possibility of him taking on some more responsibility and when he is troubled by this prospect, the authors simply encourage her to be more sympathetic and tolerant of *his* needs. By placing men's needs at the centre of the analysis, women are encouraged to put others first. The emphasis is upon what women can do to manage their partner's expectations. They are encouraged to be respectful of other's needs, gentle and not assertive, as well as – importantly – to take responsibility for others. In such texts women are thus enjoined to engage in forms of 'emotional work' (Hoschchild 2003), a practice that involves the management of one's own feelings in the private sphere. In so doing, such books reproduce an inherently gendered notion of the 'good' woman, as well as a gendered framework of emotion work.

Agency, Risk-avoidance and Prevention

Women's responsibility for acting upon the disease extends to the adoption of a series of risk-avoidance and preventative strategies. Women who already have endometriosis are told that they may be able to minimise or even resolve the disease if they avoid those things said to constitute a 'risk' to their health. In addition, self-help books target another group of subjects: those who do not even have endometriosis, but who might be able to *prevent* the disease via risk-avoidance practices. (It is not clear, of course, why women without endometriosis would be reading these books in the first place.) Despite the fact that science 'has not yet addressed prevention of endo (indeed, there's only one article on prevention of endo in the medical literature …)' (Ballweg and the Endometriosis Association 2003c: 305), self-help authors aim to encourage women to 'completely prevent the disease' and to achieve 'optimal health' (Ballweg and the Endometriosis Association 2003c: 306).

According to Alan Petersen and Iain Wilkinson (2008: 1), 'risk' has become one of the most significant 'organising principles' of our times. Everyday life is considerably influenced by the ways in which individuals think about and act towards/upon risks. The field of health care has not been immune from the increasing cultural importance of the concept of risk with risk emerging as a central concept in the sociology of health and illness in recent years (Nettleton 2006: 34). Nikolas Rose (1999: 18 cited in Robertson 2001: 299–300) has described this phenomenon as follows:

> Risk is to be managed at both collective and individual levels, minimising risk in populations as a whole, identifying and targeting high risk zones, and seeking to identify the "presymptomatic" individual at risk through the analysis of the

combinations of numerous factors, both statistically and clinically linked to the problematic conduct or pathology in question.

There are at least four separate approaches that we might use to try and explain the contemporary significance of risk (Petersen and Wilkinson 2008: 1–2; see also Mythen 2004). One approach emphasises the possibility that there is a 'psychological tendency' (Petersen and Wilkinson 2008: 1) to exaggerate the threats posed by contemporary institutions and technologies which we cannot control or influence. Another approach – arguably the most well-known approach to the study of risk – comes from the work of the German sociologist Ulrich Beck. Beck defines risk as 'a systematic way of dealing with hazards and insecurities induced and introduced by modernization itself' (1992: 21). According to Beck, risk has taken on a central place in late modern societies because we are more alert to the possibility that we are living in a dangerous world made more risky by modern technologies. Beck's perspective suggests that 'people are increasingly aware that technological hazards and industrial pollutants are drawing us to the brink of ecological catastrophe' (Petersen and Wilkinson 2008: 1).

The cultural theorist Mary Douglas argues that the increasing emphasis on risk is related to the 'rise of individualism'. Douglas' argument is not that the number or scale of *actual* risks are increasing but that because of an erosion in community, trust and tradition, we have become more anxious and 'disposed to express our concerns in terms of "risk"' (Petersen and Wilkinson 2008: 1). The fourth and final approach to the study of risk – a framework that I consider to be more valuable for present purposes – involves a more critical appraisal of risk, inspired by the work of Michel Foucault. It suggests that the centrality of risk is part of a 'governmental strategy' (Petersen and Wilkinson 2008: 2) designed to promote individual responsibility for dealing with a range of aspects of life, including the management of health concerns. As Mythen (2004: 167) explains: 'Whereas Beck postulates that awareness of manufactured threats acts as a catalyst for political reflexivity, Foucauldians accentuate the disciplinary and restrictive functions of risk'. Governmentality scholars include Lupton (2005), Robertson (2001, 2000), Petersen (1997a, 1997b) and Hughes (1997). They argue that 'risk' can operate politically, as a signifier of irresponsible citizenship and a technique of government of those citizens who 'take risks'. This approach has been used extensively in the sociological study of health and illness, including in the sociological study of genetics.

Following this governmentality approach to risk, I argue that risk-avoidance and prevention messages operate as yet another set of injunctions that are consistent with the neo-liberal philosophy of health care that has become both popular and pervasive in the West (Singleton 2003; Rimke 2000; Cheek and Rudge 1997; Petersen 1997a, 1997b). The neo-liberal philosophy sees health care as a 'private, and thus by logical inference, a self-funded affair' (Singleton 2003: 64). Messages around risk and prevention are also broadly consistent with another equally pervasive health care philosophy – that of health promotion – which includes an emphasis on disease prevention and 'healthy' living. Importantly, these ideas, insofar as they are individualised, reflect the philosophy of self-help literature itself. Self-help books are typically concerned with agitating change in the reader – part of an individualistic, aspirational 'empowerment' rhetoric that has become popular in late modernity (and which has, as I have already outlined, overlaps with the feminist movement). Neoliberalism and self-help therefore have a somewhat symbiotic relationship; a matter to which I will return later in the chapter. In the next sections, I examine four problematic aspects of these injunctions around risk avoidance and prevention. I argue, first, that risk avoidance is practically difficult, if not impossible to achieve given the abundance of risks to women's health. Secondly, I highlight some of the troublesome and gendered dimensions of calls for women to avoid risks for the benefit of others. Thirdly, I consider some of the practical limitations on women's capacity to avoid risks. And finally, I argue that it may be inherently paradoxical to speak of 'controlling' chance, which is a fundamental part of what it means to say that something is a 'risk'.

1. An Abundance of Risks

A strategy of prevention is privileged in the self-help literature, thus producing and reproducing a prevention ideology that has become prominent in late modern medicine (Nettleton 2006). The endometriosis self-help literature contains lengthy and complex lists of risks to women. For instance, women are told that a risk may be posed by exposure to certain chemicals, toxins and xeno-oestrogens (Evans 2005; Mills and Vernon 2002; Henderson and Wood 2000). They are encouraged to avoid exposure to these substances even though the relationship between such chemicals and pollutants in the environment and endometriosis is, as I noted in the earlier part of this book, uncertain (Henderson and Wood 2000: 15, 29). For example, potentially harmful substances might be found in sanitary napkins, tampons, toilet paper, facial tissues, nappies, paper plates, paper towels, coffee filters and cigarette papers (Phillips and Motta 2000: 10). Women are advised to avoid exposure to all these substances including, somehow, a multitude of products in which xeno-oestrogens might appear, such as: soaps, perfumes, pesticides, herbicides, personal care products, medicines, plastics, machines run on petroleum oil, buildings heated with petroleum oil and some clothing (Phillips and Motta 2000: 10–11).

Women are also advised to avoid dangerous substances present in many types of food (Henderson and Wood 2000: 15) and in some cases a complete change of diet is recommended (Mills and Vernon 2002: 217–18). This includes reducing intake of meat and dairy products, eating mainly organic produce, drinking water from purified sources, consuming fish only if it comes from a 'relatively clean source' such as an unpolluted lake or river, avoiding fruit or vegetables that have been sprayed with chemicals or fertilisers of any kind and avoiding processed foods, especially foods containing additives or preservatives (Mills and Vernon 2002: 217–18). Similar recommendations appear in other texts (see

Evans 2005: 256; Ballweg and the Endometriosis Association 2003; Phillips and Motta 2000: 196; Lauersen and deSwann 1988: 115–39). It is suggested that harmful substances can be found in lakes and oceans (Mills and Vernon 2002: 215) as well as in soil and water (Evans 2005: 256). The claim that substances in products, foodstuffs, soil and water may be causing illness is a very serious one. Despite the potential political, legal and ethical implications for businesses and governments, self-help books do not render this as a political, legal or ethical problem. Indeed, women are encouraged to take absolute personal responsibility for avoiding these harmful substances, even to the extent of testing soil, water and air content themselves:

> by eliminating them from your home and garden as far as possible … If you're in areas commonly sprayed with pesticides (for example golf courses), take care to keep your hands away from your mouth and wash your hands thoroughly after exposure … There are apparently over 600 known toxic waste sites in Australia, many of them in areas that are now residential housing, so if you suspect that you have only been ill since moving to a certain house, you could find out the history of your land and/or get your soil analysed. (Evans 2005: 256)

Apart from a brief reference in one text (Ballweg and the Endometriosis Association 2003), there is no suggestion that the proliferation of potentially harmful substances is, or should be, a matter for state regulation. The endometriosis self-help literature suggests that an almost limitless number of everyday substances, products and foodstuffs constitute a risk to women's health. The creation of lengthy lists of risk factors and risk-avoidance practices has a dual effect. It amplifies the range of matters with which the individual woman is to be concerned while extending the range of matters over which she will need to exert her 'authority' or 'control' if she is to manage her disease. This is highly problematic, to say the least, because women could not possibly avoid such an extensive range of risk factors. For if harmful substances are abundant and boundless, in products everywhere and in water and soil, as is claimed, the capacity of any woman to avoid exposure to all of them is necessarily limited. This suggests a fundamental incongruity in the self-help literature. Whilst women are encouraged to prevent the disease (or its recurrence) by avoiding exposure to these risks, on the one hand, the self-help literature lists risks that are in the public sphere, unregulated, seemingly infinite and, as such, practically impossible to avoid, on the other. How women live with these injunctions is something that I will come back to. Importantly, women are not only expected to avoid an abundance of risks to their health. They are also encouraged to protect others from such risks.

2. 'Prepare the Best Nest': Agency and the Maternal Self

Mary Lou Ballweg is regarded as a central figure in the worldwide endometriosis self-help movement, as I noted in Chapter 1. She devotes an entire chapter to the need for women with endometriosis to avoid risks not just for their health, but for any children they may (eventually) have. If women allow themselves to be exposed to harmful products or substances in the present, this 'may harm the health of the future child' (Ballweg and the Endometriosis Association 2003c: 310). Even women who are not yet thinking about becoming pregnant are told that they should start taking immediate action to avoid risks:

> You are your baby's first environment; just as a mother bird, you will want to prepare the best nest for your little one. You can be a good mother before conception! (Ballweg and the Endometriosis Association 2003c: 310)

'Good mothers' avoid risks before, during and after pregnancy, and manage their children's lifestyle and diets up until their teenage years (Ballweg and the Endometriosis Association 2003c). Risk avoidance is to start early: for instance, women should complete all dental work long before they fall pregnant, as some dental material is potentially toxic (2003c: 313). They are frequently advised to avoid things that might lead to their children developing the disease, in circumstances where the research remains speculative and 'preliminary'. For example, women are encouraged to exercise 'caution' about X-rays and other kinds of radiation, because it may have a causal relationship with the disease (2003c: 308). Women should also avoid dioxin-based products (such as chlorine-bleached nappies), pump breast milk between breastfeeds to avoid dioxin build-up in breast milk, 'vigilantly' watch the balance between omega-6 and omega-3 in their children's diets, give their children vitamins and minerals to boost their immune systems and use only purified water for cooking, drinking and washing food (2003c: 310–39). By suggesting that women adopt these risk-avoidance techniques, the self-help literature enacts women as principally responsible for protecting the health of their families. Moreover, the self-help literature encourages women to prevent illnesses from ever developing in future generations even though the relationship between risk-avoidance and the disease in present generations is uncertain. Whilst avoiding risks to one's own health is positioned as an individual responsibility in the self-help literature, avoiding risks for the benefit of others is positioned as a maternal responsibility. Women are called upon to avoid risks if they are '*serious* about preventing endo and related diseases in [their] children and families' (Ballweg and the Endometriosis Association 2003c: 308; my emphasis). Should her child one day develop endometriosis, the logical implication may be that the mother wasn't 'serious' enough, and that she is irresponsible and to blame.

In this sense, endometriosis self-help books do not 'reflect' existing representations of the endometriotic subject or gender – they produce and reproduce the subject, as well as gender and the feminine. In particular, the endometriotic subject is enacted as intrinsically linked to her reproductive capabilities. A central aspect of the subject is her reproductive potential and her maternal responsibilities (whether she is yet a mother or not). In this way, endometriosis self-help books enact women with endometriosis as always and inherently linked to reproduction and childbirth, whether this is of concern to her or not. Self-help books also enact 'gender' and 'femininity' in particular ways; in this example, women are reproducers and nurturers, with considerable responsibilities towards their children. Women are enacted as responsible for their offspring – not just in producing them and caring for them, but for their very constitution. In many respects, therefore, endometriosis self-help literature actually produces and reproduces a set of ideas about gender and the endometriotic subject that are already very familiar to us: women are close to nature and inherently and always linked to their reproductive facility.

3. Autonomy and the Avoidance of Risks

The endometriosis self-help literature produces its subjects as having the capacity for – or access to – extensive resources in their quest to manage the disease. The first of these has already been suggested; namely, women with endometriosis should have an enormous amount of time and energy to manage and/or avoid all of the things that constitute a risk to their health. In addition, they will need to have money. Not all women will have the financial means to eat organically, to have their soil and water tested or to buy more expensive, unbleached, unprocessed products. Whilst some authors recognise that women's options might be limited, there is little sympathy for them:

> Sometimes people say they can't afford to eat organic, and of course those in the lowest socioeconomic level can't. But I believe we really can't afford to eat any other way ... Either we pay now for high quality food that can nourish us and protect our health, or we pay later in the form of serious health problems, lost productivity, medical bills, pain, suffering, and heartache. (Ballweg and the Endometriosis Association 2003c: 328)

The other texts remain silent on these issues. They suggest that women should adopt risk-avoidance techniques but they do not acknowledge the added costs that might be involved. Similarly, the possibility that the risk-management burden may fall unevenly across the female population (by virtue of their socioeconomic status, geographic proximity to potentially harmful substances, parental or marital status and so forth) is not addressed. In ignoring the social, cultural and economic constraints on women's lives, the self-help literature produces and reproduces a highly individualised discourse of health care, exalting the individual over the social (Rimke 2000: 62). This approach generates a further contradiction in the literature.

Whilst the self-help literature promotes the notion that all women can 'stand up to the beast' (Ballweg and the Endometriosis Association 2003c: 306), the methods proffered are likely to be available to only some women and few alternatives are suggested for those who remain. Even if women could hypothetically avoid the limitless risks said to exist, it is doubtful that all women would have the time, energy and resources needed to successfully manage their health in the ways the self-help literature suggests. The rhetoric of individual 'responsibility' and 'choice' is promoted in circumstances where – by the books' own account of the disease – women may have very little capacity to act and where 'personal choice' may be restricted in a range of ways. As is the case with health promotion and the new public health, the endometriosis self-help literature operates politically in enacting the individual as the primary source of their own health, illness and wellbeing.

Endometriosis self-help literature largely neglects the material and financial constraints that will inevitably limit some women's capacity to 'autonomously' manage risks to self and others, especially with regards those risk avoidance strategies that require women to have access to money (such as purchasing organic food). Also, the literature neglects the material framework within which risks supposedly emerge: many of the apparent risks to women's health are evident in manufactured products and foodstuffs and yet the corporations who may be responsible for putting women's health 'at risk' are not challenged. The endometriosis self-help literature thus operates politically, positioning the individual, rather than the State, as both capable and culpable in disease prevention and management. In this sense, the endometriosis self-help literature endorses the ordered subjectivity and self-governing subject that is understood to be central to the neoliberal philosophy of health and illness. Paradoxically, women's ability to overcome the disease is also portrayed as being contingent upon access to extensive external resources in terms of time, money and energy. This is a fundamental contradiction in the endometriosis self-help literature: that women possess an entirely 'autonomous' self (Rose 1999) that can overcome endometriosis, at the same time as this 'autonomous' self requires material means in order to proceed.

The claim that women are 'autonomous' subjects with an unrestricted capacity for self-care is not borne out among the women that I interviewed for this research. Operating as a kind of 'moral' discourse which presumes citizens can (and will) act in 'responsible' ways, women with fewer financial resources are especially vulnerable to feelings of self-blame, anxiety and guilt when these financial constraints operate to limit their capacity for self-care. In making changes to their diets, many women had tried to eat organic produce, which can be considerably more expensive than non-organic food. Despite women's efforts to incorporate advices about toxins in foods and to prepare organic meals for themselves and their families, finances limited them. As Sally explained:

> I still feel powerless about the state of our food. If you live in a city, it's impossible to grow your own food and have access to "unpolluted" meat. If

food is organic, free-range or not tainted with chemicals – drugs, hormones, antibiotics – it is very hard to obtain and is often significantly more expensive than more readily available food. In the last couple of years, I have been able to buy free-range eggs conveniently and do so, even though they are significantly more expensive. But meat and poultry – I still buy from same shops as always. I have tried to introduce more fish and some vegetarian meals into our diet. I go through times when I'm not quite so busy – and therefore not so tired – when I cook new and varied recipes. But when I am tired, I just go back to the recipes I know well and meals become boring.

Sally's account provides a stark example of the tensions that circulate around the illusion of autonomous selfhood. Moreover, Sally's capacity to avoid environmental toxins is also limited because she lives in a city and cannot easily grow her own food. Even then she does not have the energy to prepare a diverse range of meals.

Similar themes recurred throughout my interviews. Hannah, for example, spent $200 a month on her health, explaining that some 'weeks I didn't have enough money for essentials like food and bills'. Another woman, Wanda, was unemployed and receiving a disability pension because of the severity of her condition. She felt she had 'no other option' but to try and avoid things that posed a risk to her health as risk-avoidance was 'the right thing to do'. Being on welfare, however, meant that her options were limited:

> I was willing to try acupuncture but could not afford it. And there was also – I can't think of the name – but it's like a herbalist who looks into the eyes and sees what's wrong [with your health]. But I also couldn't afford that … it all costs money, so really it's a crock of shit. I went to a naturopath once. They wanted me to take a herbal treatment every week. It would cost $80. Every week. There was no way I could afford it. So I never went back. I felt really shit and I've had to try hard not to dwell on it.

Instead of going to acupuncture and the naturopath, Wanda did what she could, avoiding those risks that did not require her to spend money, like limiting her intake of alcohol and coffee. Still, she 'felt really shit' about not being able to do more and blamed herself for not being responsible enough. This sense of self-blame was also articulated by Alexis, who struggled financially. Whilst she was acutely aware of risks and risk-avoidance practices, she could not afford to undertake all of them. Despite her attempts to manage her health and eat 'properly', Alexis was unable to do everything she felt she should be doing. She explained:

> I have tried to do lots of reading and things. And a good friend of mine, a couple of times has recommended a naturopath but I haven't got around to saving up the money and going, which is really terrible. And it's bad because you think

that your health is obviously something really important and something worth investing in and taking seriously ... And it's terrible, but it tended to be an issue of money. These last few months have been the first time in years that I have been working full-time and that's been two part-time things. I've generally been on my lowly arts manager salary and living alone and sort of making ends meet. And I often sit back and reflect on what a terrible person this makes me, because I am not putting my health first.

Despite the obvious impact of Alexis' material circumstances on her capacity to take up risk avoidance and preventative strategies, she did not perceive those material circumstances to be the factor that inhibited her. She sees *herself* as the problem. Alexis' fear that she had been a 'terrible person' for not 'putting her health first' suggests a profound sense that, as a choosing subject, she should have had absolute control over the course of her own care.

In a classic statement on the divisive consequences of an individualised discourse of health living and health promotion, Robin Bunton and Roger Burrows (1995: 211) argued:

> Whilst some people may be able to pay for cosmetic surgery, others have to wait for unacceptably long periods just for routine relief from pain and other obstacles to their daily lives. Whilst some can afford to choose extra virgin olive oil and fresh vegetables, others have to sleep in cardboard boxes on the streets and eat what food they can get.

Forms of 'healthy' living that are materialised in self-help literature are simply not open to everyone. As such, discourses of risk and risk-avoidance may be a catalyst for women (especially women with fewer financial means) to blame themselves for developing endometriosis. Several commentators have drawn attention to processes of self-blame in relation to health. In a society that expects their ostensibly 'autonomous' citizens to take care of their health as a private concern, those who do not do 'everything' they can for their health become 'irresponsible citizens' (Rimke 2000). This has been variously described as a breach of a 'social contract of health' (Cheek and Rudge 1997) and at the individual level it is experienced as a form of personal or 'moral failure' (Petersen 1997b). Both Wanda and Alexis viewed themselves as failures: Wanda 'felt really shit' and 'tried hard not to dwell' on her failure and Alexis saw herself as a 'terrible person' for not putting her health 'first'. In so doing, these women failed to behave like 'proper' citizens in a society that has become increasingly attached to the notion that healthy living is a signifier of responsible citizenship (Rimke 2000). Although self-help books are not necessarily responsible for how these women ultimately act and/or view themselves, they do very little to persuade women otherwise. Indeed, as I have argued, self-help books usually actively encourage women to see the disease as their responsibility.

4. Controlling Risks: A Paradox?

In recent years, risk has emerged as an important concept in the field of health and illness (Nettleton 2006: 34). Sociologists have been interested in exploring a very broad range of factors associated with this field, including how health risks are perceived, negotiated, 'amplified' and calculated. There has been a recent and dramatic increase in the number of studies that examine how the media portrays risks (Kitzinger 1999: 56). Within this broader subset of interest, several scholars have explored how health risks are communicated to publics (e.g. Petersen 2005; Lupton 2004; Slovic 1986). Principally, such studies involve analyses of how the print and television media communicate risks. Much of this work is underpinned by a realist understanding of risks; analyses of the extent to which a given text 'amplifies' a risk, for instance, will be necessarily predicated on an understanding of the risk as both stable and quantifiable. For the reasons I have already outlined, however, this is not a position that I consider can be sustained. I am more interested in the way that self-help literature functions to *materialise* risk. It goes without saying, then, that whether or not the endometriosis risks are 'real' is not my present concern. As Mary Douglas (1990: 8) once said, the argument 'is not about the reality of the dangers, but about how they are politicized'.

According to Deborah Lupton 'risk' is a concept with several different meanings, depending on who is using the term. The proliferation of usages of the term in both vernacular and professional applications means that its meanings are both complex and confusing (2005: 422). Traditionally, risk was a neutral term, used principally in the field of mathematics to denote the probability or statistical likelihood of a given event occurring (Lupton 2005: 423). Common dictionary definitions of 'risk' retain some of this early meaning, indicating that 'risk' involves an element of 'chance', or 'hazard'. Mary Douglas (1990) argues that risk has become a value-laden term signifying 'danger'. But she is careful not to conflate the two terms. Risk continues to be invoked in certain circumstances because it means both 'danger' and 'chance': 'danger would have been the right word, but plain danger does not have the aura of science or afford the pretension of a possible precise calculation' (Douglas 1990: 4). For the purposes of my argument, I am interested in the fact that risk is usually taken to reference the 'chance' that a given event – such as the development of a disease – will transpire. Women are encouraged to guard against such risks in endometriosis self-help texts, and to 'stand up to the beast' (Ballweg and the Endometriosis Association 2003c: 306). This can be achieved, it seems, through risk-avoidance.

Given that endometriosis is enacted as a disease of risks in the self-help literature and given that 'risk' means exposure to the possibility of something occurring, the notion that women can control a disease (that is, control possibility) seems strangely paradoxical. Of course, it may be possible to minimise exposure to risks (and thus, the possibility of disease developing or spreading) through, for instance, the introduction of organic produce into one's diet. But it is a logical confusion to speak of controlling the disease when that control rests upon avoidance of exposure to chance. The endometriosis self-help literature glosses over these tensions and constitutes risks as containable and controllable, in keeping with the modernist tenets of rationality and mastery. The prospect of the disease's occurrence or recurrence is depicted as both rationally calculable and objectively knowable, in contrast to most medical literature. In this sense self-help books are underpinned by what Robert Castel (1991: 289) has called the 'grandiose technocratic rationalising dream of absolute control of the accidental'. This is a major ethical and political problem and raises questions about the responsibilities of authors in producing such accounts of the disease.

Conclusion

According to Jackie Stacey, the post-Enlightenment epoch is characterised by:

> the desire for mastery. It is the desire to see, to know and to control. It is the desire to fix meaning and to make outcomes predictable. It is the desire to prove that one has power over disease, the body and the emotions. (1997: 238)

Self-help literature both reflects and reproduces these key Enlightenment ideals, by suggesting that it is possible to understand and conquer disease and the body: to 'master' the seemingly 'mysterious' and 'enigmatic' features of endometriosis. In self-help literature, the central resource in mastering disease is not the doctor, nor the expert authors of the books: it is the sufferers themselves. Women are positioned as possessing an inherent capacity to overcome endometriosis, but also an obligation – to self and others – to take action. In this sense, self-help books enact women as simultaneously agentive and obliged to exercise their agency in ways that might positively impact upon their disease and those around them. The notion that health and illness can be controlled is a form of what Robert Crawford (1980) has called 'healthism'. Healthism suggests that an 'individual has choice in preserving his or her physical capacity from the event of disease' (Petersen 1997b: 198). Although 'moral theories of illness have always held a firm place in traditional belief systems, across cultures and over time' (Galvin 2002: 109), the idea that 'health is something which lies within the control of the individual' (Nettleton 1997: 208) has become increasingly prominent in late-modern, Western discursive contexts. Endometriosis self-help books undoubtedly reflect this trend and work to reinforce it, mainly through the way they perform disease, agency and the disease-subject relation. Importantly, however, these books represent an example of the way that practices that are broadly compatible with healthism often also invoke and produce gendered notions of agency and responsibility with regards to self, body, emotions and others.

The enactment of women as inherently masterful and responsible for disease management and prevention depends partly upon a configuration of endometriosis as a largely stable and coherent object. This depiction of the disease is at odds with the way some medical literature enacts it. It is also at odds with traditional conceptions of women's agency where women figure as passive, vulnerable and close to nature. The way that self-help books enact the disease and its subjects is likely to (at least partly) be a function of the expectations that surround the genre. Authors may assume, for example, that readers want self-help books to be 'positive', 'motivational', 'inspiring' and 'empowering', so that they are compelled to draw the subjects therein in just this way. The form and content of the books that I have analysed in this chapter are likely, therefore, to respond to the assumptions and expectations of the genre – where an agentive subject is constituted as capable of bringing a troublesome but coherent object under their control. In so doing, the authors reinforce the agentive and masterful subject as a key 'feature' of the genre. I would also argue that the abundance of injunctions articulated in self-help literature are a product, in part, of the many uncertainties and competing claims about the disease. In other words, because it is not clear what causes the disease, the net for health self-management ends up being cast particularly widely. In this way, *uncertainty, confusion and mess is productive.* It may be productive in terms of agency, as well, perhaps, for the materiality of the disease more broadly. As regards the former, although individual readers will undoubtedly engage with this literature in diverse ways, there is always the possibility that women will come away with a heightened and potentially problematic understanding of their responsibilities and agency vis-à-vis the disease. This is because, as I have already argued, self-help books render endometriosis as a manifestation, variously, of a disordered or improperly realised agency, whether through disordered habits of consumption or an inappropriate relationship to one's own 'femininity'. Endometriosis is ultimately a function of the woman herself. Self-help books therefore work to enact the disease and agency in ways that are both largely familiar and ethically and politically unsound.

Given these findings, I want to conclude my analysis in this chapter with a set of questions about responsibility in self-help – but not in such a way as to again imply that it is the patients themselves who are responsible for the disease and its management. Rather, I wonder what might be the responsibilities of the *authors* of these books and others involved in their production? Might we consider their agency as – at times – inappropriately realised and disordered, through its role in the ethics and politics of gender and disease? As I explained at the outset of this chapter, following Law (2002), writing is always and already politics, and is one of the main ways by which the world is performed. Because of this, of course, new versions of disease, subjectivity and agency are always possible. My approach in this chapter, as another form of writing, is no different; it is also a kind of politics, performing disease, agency and responsibility in ways that I hope will challenge conventional understandings of self-help literature. The authors of future self-help books have the opportunity – indeed, I suggest, the *responsibility* – to approach the disease and its subjects differently. Moreover, to the extent that endometriosis may actually be a function of women's engagement with medical treatment, environment, risk factors and so on, self-help literature is uniquely positioned to shape the very materiality of the epidemic 'itself'.

Self-help authors could approach this task in various ways. For example, future work could engage much more critically with the notion that women are obliged to manage and govern risks to their own health and the health of others. There could be a more explicit engagement with the agency and responsibility of those within biomedicine, but also others, including the State, to whom questions about chemical and environmental regulation might be put. If hormones present in food and other products are implicated in any way in the development of the disease, why don't self-help authors engage more directly with the manufacturers of food, or the regulators of food, about their responsibilities to the public? Surely there is a need to look more carefully at the agency and responsibility of various key stakeholders in this respect. Self-help books could also be more explicit about the possible limitations of women's agency, rather than producing women as autonomous selves capable of mastering their illness. In this sense, self-help authors might look to examine (and thus, enact) women's agency in ways that align more closely with how women understand themselves as agents. This could be done through engagement with research which has already examined these questions, including my own work on women's compliance with injunctions to self-care (Seear 2009d). As I have explained in this chapter, women with endometriosis typically understand themselves as agentive, but view their agency as restricted in several important ways, including materially. Self-help authors would do well to engage with the diversity of women's experiences and to acknowledge the political and ethical dimensions of constituting agency and responsibility in this regard. This, of course, is a fine balance; I understand that many authors will be concerned to try and actively revive women's agency through the pages of self-help books, but they must be careful that in so doing they do not reach too far the other way. Although this is a challenging task, the stakes of doing nothing – or of continuing to get it wrong – are very high indeed. For women like Wanda, who felt exhausted and 'shit' about herself for not complying with these messages, there is a need for urgent reflection, and for more care and attention in the messages distributed to women living with this disease.

Chapter 4

The Typical Patient Profile:
On Treatment and the
Constitution of Subjects

The question of "the subject" is crucial for politics.

(Butler, 1990: 2)

One of the most persistent features of the last 150 years of endometriosis medicine has been the central role of the endometriotic 'subject' in medical and popular accounts of the disease. Although ideas about the subject have changed over time, endometriosis has frequently been positioned as a disease peculiar to affluent, white, career-oriented women. Individually and collectively, women with endometriosis, it has been claimed, have certain personality traits: they tend to be perfectionists, who are intelligent, anxious and egocentric. Consequently, biomedicine has approached the diagnosis and treatment of women with endometriosis with this 'typical patient profile' in mind. Historically, for instance, some medical literature asserted that poor, non-Caucasian or childbearing women were, at best, highly unlikely to develop endometriosis. Doctors were thus encouraged to discount endometriosis as a possible diagnosis, regardless of the symptoms presented, in any women who did not fit these classifications. Almost undoubtedly, then, some women will have experienced delays to diagnosis (or perhaps they were never diagnosed) unless, in the eyes of their treating physician, they fitted the profile, which is to say that they were classed as 'white', 'affluent', 'intelligent', or 'career-oriented', however these categories were constituted. As well as bearing upon diagnosis, the *treatment* of women with endometriosis was tied to this 'typical patient profile'. In some medical literature, for example, the most appropriate way to treat intelligent or career-oriented women with endometriosis was to discourage them from the pursuit of education or careers and to promote childbirth, childrearing, breastfeeding and the role of housewife, in the alternative. Importantly, the pursuit of childbirth and childrearing were not advanced along purely ideological grounds (even if such a distinction could be maintained); indeed, medical literature was replete with claims that pregnancy was a medical cure for endometriosis, a notion that still persists today.

The aim of this chapter is twofold. Taking the question of treatment as its referent, this chapter critically interrogates the 'typical patient profile', and the oft-repeated claim that women with endometriosis, both individually and collectively, share several attributes and traits. As an associated (but no less vital) task, the chapter critically explores what happens in and through endometriosis treatment – a realm, I argue, that is highly politicised and ethically charged. Following the work of feminist theorist Judith Butler and later, Karen Barad, this chapter asks: How is the 'typical patient' intra-actively constituted through treatment? Taking as my critical starting point theoretical challenges to the notion of the subject as foundational, or as anterior to social relations (e.g. Barad 2003, 2007; Butler 1993) this chapter challenges the notion that the endometriotic subject and/or the 'typical patient' exists prior to her management through biomedicine. The chapter also considers some of the ways that treatment performs spatio-temporal arrangements, and the significance of time, in particular, for the materialisation of endometriosis as epidemic. The chapter begins with a detailed discussion of feminist theory on the subject and the significance of this work for understanding the politics and ethics of health care practices. After this, I outline the main approaches to the treatment of endometriosis. I then consider how two treatment regimens manifest in endometriosis: the first being injunctions to treat the disease through pregnancy, and the second through the administration of hormonal therapies. I look at how each of these relates to understandings about the behavioural traits and attributes that women with endometriosis, as a collective, supposedly exhibit. I argue that both forms of treatment produce and reproduce the 'typical endometriotic patient' – a subject that is assumed to pre-exist her diagnosis and enrolment in treatment. I also consider the enactment of women as non-compliant patients. This is a highly politicised subject position with major implications for women, but also, as we will see, for the emergence of endometriosis as a modern epidemic.

The Question of the Subject

One of the central organising principles of Western, post-Enlightenment societies is the notion of subjects as foundational, unified and stable. As the feminist theorist and quantum physicist Karen Barad explains:

> Liberal social theories and theories of scientific knowledge alike owe much to the idea that the world is composed of individuals – presumed to exist before the law, or the discovery of the law – awaiting/inviting representation. The idea that beings exist as individuals with inherent attributes, anterior to their representation, is a metaphysical presupposition that underlies the belief in political, linguistic, and epistemological forms of representationalism. Or, to put the point the other way around, representationalism is the belief in the ontological distinction between representations and that which they purport to represent; in particular, that which is represented is held to be independent of all practices of representing. (2003: 803–4)

The ideas associated with representationalism have been the subject of extensive critique in recent years, in fields as diverse as feminist theory, race and cultural studies and queer theory. Two of the most prominent theorists to pose a challenge to these ideas are the French philosopher Michel Foucault and the feminist and queer theorist Judith Butler. (For a more detailed discussion on both, see my earlier work with Suzanne Fraser.) Drawing upon Foucault's configuration of power-knowledge and the significance of this for subjectivity, Butler explains the problems with representationalism in this way:

> Juridical notions of power appear to regulate political life in purely negative terms – that is, through the limitation, prohibition, regulation, control, and even "protection" of individuals related to that political structure through the contingent and retractable operation of choice. But the subjects regulated by such structures are, by virtue of being subjected to them, formed, defined and reproduced in accordance with the requirements of those structures. (1990: 2–3)

In other words, as Foucault explains in 'Two Lectures':

> The individual is not to be conceived as a sort of elementary nucleus, a primitive atom, a multiple and inert material on which power comes to fasten or against which it happens to strike, and in so doing subdues or crushes individuals. In fact, it is already one of the prime effects of power that certain bodies, certain gestures, certain discourses, certain desires, come to be identified and constituted as individuals. The individual, that is, is not the vis-à-vis of power; it is, I believe, one of its prime effects. The individual is an effect of power and at the same time, or precisely to the extent to which it is that effect, it is the element of its articulation. The individual which power has constituted is at the same time its vehicle. (1980b: 98)

For present purposes, the significance of Butler's work lies in her engagement with the role of practices in materialising sex and gender. Seeking to move away from essentialist and determinist accounts of sex/gender that emphasise matter as wholly determinative, Butler instead engages with the significance of practices in surfacing bodies, subjects and subjectivities (as I flagged briefly in the opening chapter). In *Gender Trouble* (1990) for instance, Butler introduces the concept of gender performativity as a means of understanding gender 'not as a thing or a set of free-floating attributes, not as an essence – but rather as a "doing"' (Barad 2003: 808), through emphasising gender as 'a kind of becoming or activity', as 'an incessant and repeated action of some sort' (Butler 1990: 112). Later in her invaluable text *Bodies That Matter* (1993), Butler expanded further on the question of the production of subjects.[1] In one of her most famous passages, she writes:

---

1 Although these are ideas that I have engaged with in my earlier work on hepatitis C, together with Suzanne Fraser (2011), they also bear upon the present discussion, and are worth considering once more.

> This exclusionary matrix by which subjects are formed thus requires the
> simultaneous production of a domain of abject beings, those who are not yet
> subjects, but who form the constitutive outside to the domain of the subject. The
> abject designates here precisely those "unlivable" and "uninhabitable" zones of
> social life which are nevertheless densely populated by those who do not enjoy
> the status of the subject, but whose living under the sign of the "unlivable" is
> required to circumscribe the domain of the subject. (1993: 3)

Here, then, subjects are understood to manifest through processes of exclusion
and inclusion. Abject subjects emerge as the counterpoint to subjects, in much
the same way that other binaries (nature/culture, order/chaos, authenticity/falsity)
emerge through one another, as I discussed in Chapter 1.[2] According to Butler,
subjects surface through practices and methods of exclusion and inclusion. The
materialisation of subjects is always already dependent upon the concurrent
assembly of that subject's antithesis – what Butler calls 'the domain of the abject'.
As she explains:

> In this sense, then, the subject is constituted through the force of exclusion and
> abjection, one which produces a constitutive outside to the subject, an abjected
> outside, which is, after all, "inside" the subject as its own founding repudiation.
> (Butler 1993: 3)

The abject does not enjoy the status of the subject against whom it is produced
through the forces of exclusion and abjection. Instead, the abject inhabits the
unlivable and uninhabitable zones of social life, while the subject inhabits livable
social zones. Importantly, just as the categories and domains of the subject and the
abject do not pre-exist their materialisation through processes of exclusion and
inclusion, neither do those 'things' with which each is materially and symbolically
associated. So, to the extent that the subject is associated with autonomy
and freedom, for example, the meaning of 'freedom' is something that itself
materialises in connection with the materialisation of the subject. These emerge
in a continual process of mutual production. Crucially, each materialisation of the
subject simultaneously works to materialise what the subject is not – or, in other
words, to produce the domain of the abject. Subject and abject depend upon each
other, with these mutual dependencies and movements functioning ontologically
and politically, as one figure in every binary pairing is devalued and subordinate,
the other is valorised and superior. In this sense, the constitution of subjects is
always and already a political and ethical process; it is why, according to Butler
(1990: 2), 'the question of "the subject" is crucial for politics'.

---

2   For more, see, for example, Derrida (1976), Grosz (1989).

The Question of Matter

Although Butler denies that 'the body is simply linguistic stuff' (1993: 68), she has often been accused of overplaying the roles of language, culture and discourse, to the relative neglect of matter, nature and the non-human (for a discussion, see, for example, Barad 2007: 61–4; Kirby 2006). Concerns about the extent to which the performative/discursive turn engages with materiality have been explored and developed most completely in recent years by Karen Barad. Her work (2007, 1998, 2003) on agency and subjectivity offers, as we shall see, invaluable insights of direct relevance to the treatment of women with endometriosis. According to Barad, the problem with some recent work – including work in feminist theory – is that:

> Language has been granted too much power. The linguistic turn, the semiotic turn, the interpretative turn, the cultural turn: it seems that at every turn lately every "thing" – even materiality – is turned into a matter of language or some other form of cultural representation ... Language matters. Discourse matters. Culture matters. There is an important sense in which the only thing that does not seem to matter anymore is matter. (2003: 801)

She argues that although language and culture have been 'granted their own agency and historicity', matter has come to figure as 'passive and immutable' (2003: 801). We need to be careful, Barad argues, not to figure matter 'as merely an end product rather than an active factor in further materializations', because to do so 'is to cheat matter out of the fullness of its capacity' (2003: 810).

Barad's way of working through these issues is to propose a posthumanist performativity: a set of theoretical concepts that, taken together, is grounded in the fundamental notion that subjects and objects do not pre-exist, but are constituted through various practices, including human and non-human realms. Barad, following the quantum physicist Niels Bohr, speaks of objects and subjects as 'phenomena'; they are constituted, that is, through processes of what she calls 'intra-action'. As she explains:

> The notion of intra-action is a key element of my agential realist framework. The neologism "intra-action" *signifies the mutual constitution of entangled agencies*. That is, in contrast to the usual "interaction", which assumes that there are separate individual agencies that proceed their interaction, the notion of intra-action recognizes that distinct agencies do not precede, but rather emerge through, their intra-action. (2007: 33)

Importantly, Barad extends these observations to space and time, which, she argues, must also be considered as constituted as part of the 'dynamics of intra-activity' (2007: 180). Rejecting the idea of time as an 'exterior parameter', or space as a 'container' within which things take place, Barad makes the point that 'space, time and matter are mutually constituted through the dynamics of iterative intra-activity. The space-time manifold is iteratively (re)configured in terms of how material-discursive practices come to matter' (2007: 181). In this sense, Barad sees time and space, among other things, as the products of one another – as *co-constituted phenomena*. Such radical re-workings of material-discursive relations lend to new ways of understanding causality.

One pertinent illustration of how ideas such as these might be applied to the politics of health care can be found in the work of Suzanne Fraser (2006). Fraser's work considers the constitution of subjects via the highly politicised practice of methadone maintenance treatment in Australia. Through focusing on the discrete event of subjects regularly queuing at clinics throughout the Australian state of New South Wales for methadone dosing, Fraser considers how the subject category of the 'drug addict' materialises via the spatio-temporal arrangement of methadone dosing within which subjects are treated:

> Although clinics tend to operate as if they are observing and treating clients who have pre-existing attributes (in Barad's terms, relata), they can also be viewed as co-constituting clients through a process of intra-action. In other words, the client and the queue co-construct each other. The programme does not take pre-formed "addicts", observe their behaviour and then treat them to produce a reliable outcome that can be understood as the reproducible effect of the programme. Rather, clients, themselves already multiply co-constituted phenomena, intra-act with the chronotope of methadone maintenance treatment (that is, the queue – itself also always already multiply co-constituted). In the process, both the client and the queue impact on each other, reproducing each other differently. Thus, the specific forms of time and space at work at the clinic help shape the client and his or her experiences, rather than simply acting as a conduit for these experiences. (2006: 199)

In other words, the subject does not pre-exist the process of queueing but is enacted through it, as well as the materiality of drugs and methadone: the 'chronotope of the clinic acts as much to produce particular kinds of clients as it does to treat them' (2006: 200). Importantly, Fraser goes beyond conventional analyses that might assume space and time as fixed, given or prior, and understands them as being both co-constituted through and co-constituting the subjects and objects that make up methadone maintenance treatment. Nicole Vittelone (2011) has also recognised the utility of Barad's work for studies of drug use, particularly in Barad's refusal to distinguish between the human and non-human in the co-constitution of phenomena. Interested specifically in the operation of the syringe in injecting drug use, Vitellone argues that the syringe needs to be reconceptualised as 'an object that is fully alive to the event at hand', as opposed to 'a dead device that simply facilitates action between humans' (2011: 201). Although the work of both Fraser and Vitellone deals with a seemingly very different sphere (drug use-treatment) to the one in question here, each offers a pertinent reminder of double significance. First, they remind us of the now ineffaceable point that both subjects and objects are not anterior to social relations. And secondly, any investigation of phenomena must work to first shake itself free from approaches that operate to render matter inert or lifeless. In what follows, I consider how these ideas might be extended to an analysis of women's experiences of endometriosis treatment. With limited exceptions (e.g. Cox 2003a, 2003b), women's experiences with endometriosis treatment have not often been explored in the academic literature.[3] This chapter engages explicitly with women's accounts of treatment through an analysis of interviews with women who have been diagnosed with the condition. Following Barad, my concern is with the specific question of what becomes-in-the-world through the phenomenon of endometriosis treatment. The key focus of the chapter is upon the constitution of subjects through treatment. In what follows, I want to challenge the idea that endometriosis medicine merely treats a pre-existing category of subjects that we might call 'typical patients' or, alternatively, 'women with endometriosis' (phrases that are both integral to endometriosis medicine). Instead, I argue, treatment regimens are one of the principal means by which endometriotic subjects are constituted. Treatment makes, as I shall argue, the very subjects it purports to treat; the typical patients, that is, that are first profiled, then diagnosed and finally, treated, through contemporary biomedicine. As part of this process, treatment intra-actively co-constitutes time and space, a crucial component in the materialisation of the epidemic. In all of these respects, treatment needs to be understood as a dynamic process that participates in fundamental ways to the making of the epidemic. I conclude the chapter with a consideration of what my analysis means for approaches to the management of the disease.

The Typical Patient Profile

The question of subjecthood is central to endometriosis medicine for a range of reasons. The field of endometriosis medicine as a whole has long been characterised by speculation about the *specific types of women* that are most likely to develop the disease. My own examination of the history of medical literature on endometriosis leaves no doubt that biomedicine has consistently assumed one of its central tasks to be the diagnosis and treatment – not just of women, but of *certain kinds of women*. Crucially, these subjects are understood to pre-exist the biomedical encounter. Perhaps the best exemplar of this notion is the oft-discussed 'typical patient profile', an omnipresent concept in endometriosis medicine that is

---

3   To some extent, Ella Shohat's (1998) work on laser laparoscopy does engage with the question of treatment, but her focus differs markedly from mine here, in that she was principally concerned with how the laparoscope is represented, and how this functions more broadly in configuring the subject and medicine.

simultaneously pervasive and persistent. Importantly, the 'typical patient profile' is not static; indeed, it is dynamic, fluid and changeable. When I talk about the typical patient profile, then, I refer not to a fixed notion of who the endometriotic subject is, but to *a set of practices* through which the subject is constituted and re-constituted across time. Although her characteristics may change, as will the language utilised to describe her, the typical patient has a set of relatively constant features.

The most prominent version of the typical patient profile involves the career-oriented subject. It is difficult to pinpoint its exact origins, nor when the term was first introduced, but a review of the medical literature confirms that endometriosis was being widely touted as a 'career women's disease' by at least the 1970s. The phrase was frequently used in medical texts throughout that decade and the next, along with clinical studies (e.g. Lauersen and deSwann 1988; Lewis, Comite, Mallouh, et al. 1987; Lauersen and Whitney 1977; Chalmers 1975; Kistner 1971). Put simply, the 'typical' endometriosis patient was one who worked, or who had worked. In this sense, endometriosis was thought to strike only those women who had prioritised a career over family. (By extension, then, the typical patient profile positioned career and family as mutually exclusive.)

Another typical patient profile constituted women with endometriosis as being 'meticulous in their personal habits' and the disease was said to rarely occur in 'obese or sloppy women' (Older 1984: 137). In an oft-repeated account of the 'typical patient profile' as it manifested during the 1970s, the gynaecologist Robert Kistner explained:

> It has been suggested that a specific body type and psychic demeanor are frequently found. The patient is said to be mesomorphic but underweight, overanxious, intelligent, egocentric and a perfectionist. These characteristics represent a personality pattern in which marriage and childbearing are likely to be deferred and therefore predispose to prolonged periods of uninterrupted ovulation. (1971: 441)

At the same time, Kistner also claimed that endometriosis was 'not common in the Negro *[sic]* and seems to be found more among women of the higher socio-economic groups. As such, it has been correlated with delayed or deferred motherhood' (1971: 441).[4] Typical endometriosis patients are tense perfectionists: 'that type of individual who simply has to clean out the ashtrays all the time' (Kistner quoted in Older 1984: 135). In this version of the typical patient profile, Joe Vincent Meigs' ideas about nature, culture and the body – discussed in Chapter 1 – can be seen to

---

4   As I have already discussed, endometriosis was long considered to be a disease unique to white women. Endometriosis is now diagnosed amongst women of all races and ethnic groups, although some research still suggests that it is less prevalent in African-American women than Caucasian women (e.g. Missmer, Hankinson, Spiegelman, et al. 2004).

surface once again; specifically, the idea that motherhood is a natural and normal function of women and that endometriosis occurs only in those women who have 'delayed' or 'deferred' that role. Moreover, the notion of pregnancy as a moral imperative amongst women, prominent throughout Meigs' work, was reiterated.[5]

Assertions about the typical patient profile, at least in some quarters, were drawn from clinical experience. Writing in the 1980s, Lauersen and deSwann claimed, for example: 'that nearly 95 percent of endometriosis patients are women under extreme stress who work or who have worked' (Lauersen and deSwann 1988: 7).[6] Their explanation of the relationship between endometriosis and the 'deferment' of childbearing is illustrative:

> In simpler cultures where age-old, traditional women's roles are still abided by, women bear their first child at an earlier age. They then breast-feed their child, conceive a second child, and the cycle begins again. Over their life-spans, women who have borne children at a younger age, or who eventually have larger families, are found to be less frequent victims of endometriosis ... Over the last twenty years, however, as personal achievement for women in developed countries has become more defined by professional gains than by exacting and rearing a family, the incidence of endometriosis has increased. (Lauersen and deSwann 1988: 20)

Lauersen and deSwann's account enacts at least two subject positions: the 'modern' woman, who prioritises personal interests over public ones, and 'traditional' women, who prioritise family over career. Accounts such as this one function in at least three ways: working to produce, reproduce and valorise traditional women's roles within society, and, at the same time, to devalue those modern women who do not so conform. The ethical and political significance of enactments such as these is a matter to which I will return later in the chapter.

The 'typical patient profile' – however it looks at any given point in time – has a crucial relationship with ways of managing the disease. Historically, for example, it was common for physicians to suggest that marriage and/or pregnancy would cure the disease at those times that career-orientation was understood to be

---

5 Sexual intercourse was also a moral imperative. Comments made by Dr Mary Lou Hollis are typical of this attitude, with the suggestion that complaints of painful intercourse were simply 'a nice protection for some women who do not want children' (Hollis cited in Capek 2000: 360).

6 When Lauersen and deSwann talk about 'work', presumably they mean only *paid* work. This is an extremely narrow definition of work that fails to account for the whole range of human experience, including unpaid or involuntary work and, most notably, childcare or housework as forms of work. Moreover, implicit in Lauersen and deSwann's comments is the notion that forms of unpaid work, such as childcare, are not likely to cause stress and, consequently, the development of endometriosis. An alternative interpretation is that the impact of their descriptors may create a divide between acceptable forms of work (housework and childcare) and unacceptable forms (paid employment).

a predisposing factor to its development (e.g. Lauersen and deSwann 1988: 20; Lauersen and Whitney 1977: 334; Chalmers 1975: 117; Kistner 1971: 444). This has been a long-standing practice among physicians, extending as far back at least as Joe Vincent Meigs, who exhorted doctors to encourage early marriage and frequent childbearing. Even Robert Kistner, who took a special interest in endometriosis and encouraged physicians to see it as a 'crippling' and serious condition, saw endometriosis as principally a condition of fertility. His primary concern was that endometriosis prevented 'the fulfilment of [women's] marital potential' (Kistner 1971: 444). In the fourth edition of *Operative Gynecology* a range of possible treatments were described but it was argued: 'Since endometriosis is usually a benign process becoming quiescent with the menopause, its presence does not necessarily constitute an indication for treatment' unless, perhaps, the patient desires to preserve her 'childbearing function' (TeLinde and Mattingly 1970: 217). Even as physicians began to question the idea that endometriosis was a career women's disease,[7] the idea that marriage and/or pregnancy may cure it persisted (Rhodes 1996: 106). So, as Missmer and Cramer (2003: 15) claim, for example, there could be a link between pregnancy and the disease through the decreased exposure to menstrual blood:

> It is also reasonable to propose that delayed childbearing also could be a cause of endometriosis. Although avoided menstruation is one explanation for a protective effect of childbearing, it should also be appreciated that permanent cervical dilation occurs with labor and delivery, possibly reducing the resistance to menstrual flow and decreasing the likelihood of retrograde menstruation.

The 'career women's' designation has been criticised in feminist, medical and self-help literature in recent years (e.g. Carpan 2003). The 'typical patient' appears to look a little different over the last decade, as does the language that is used to describe her. In a 2005 paper, 'Who gets endometriosis?', Kennedy explained changes in the field in this way:

> It is widely believed that endometriosis occurs more commonly in middle-aged, upper-class, ambitious, white women. However, there is no evidence to support these beliefs. The stereotype probably demonstrates only that such women have greater access to medical care and a laparoscopic diagnosis. (2005: 18)

---

7   Despite the fact that changes were occurring in the medical profession's attitudes towards the 'typical patient profile', literature from the late 1980s continued to perpetuate connections between personality, career choice and the condition. For example, Boling, Abbasi, Ackerman, et al. (1988: 49) noted: 'The patients tend to be mostly professional, perfectionists with a desire to excel. As such, the time lost from work makes a significant difference in their economic, physical and psychological well-being.'

Later, in the same paper, Kennedy detailed the latest manifestation of the typical patient profile, one that pointedly invokes the concept of 'risk', as opposed to personality types described by Kistner more than 30 years earlier:

> However, some women undoubtedly are more likely to develop endometriosis and the factors contributing to that increased risk are the subject of much research interest at the moment ... In many studies, the risk of endometriosis seems clearly related to an increased exposure to menstruation. Thus, a shorter menstrual cycle length (≤27 days), longer duration of flow (>1 week) and reduced parity have all been identified as risk factors, as well as a need for double protection (i.e. pads and tampons) related to the heaviness of the flow. These data have been used to support the idea that endometriosis arises because of retrograde menstruation. They are also consistent with the finding that endometriosis is commonly found in women with Müllerian anomalies, e.g. congenital absence of the cervix, because of the increased backflow. (2005: 18–19)

Clearly, then, women with endometriosis continue to be understood as exhibiting a set of characteristics that is inherent to them individually. As a collective, they are unique, with characteristics consistent across the endometriotic population. This notion – that women with endometriosis possess consistent, anterior and stable features of certain kinds – appears right across the spectrum of endometriosis medicine. The scouring work of epidemiologists, for instance, both assumes and reproduces 'women with endometriosis' as a largely homogeneous group, through seeking out patterns and connections regarding the *kinds of women* that are likely to develop the disease. In medical education and through medical textbooks, doctors are taught that women with endometriosis are likely to behave in certain ways, exhibit specific qualities, possess particular traits and are thus at an elevated level of 'risk'. These ideas make their way into clinics, as physicians are encouraged to suspect endometriosis if any woman presenting with certain gynaecological symptoms also appears to be the *kind of woman* that fits the profile – first, that of the career woman, now that of the subject at 'risk' – to which they have been exposed. In all of these ways, endometriosis medicine appears to be concerned with identifying pre-existing patterns and connections. A skilled physician is one that can join up all of the dots, and treat the subject accordingly. In the next sections, I challenge the pre-existence of the typical patient through a consideration of women's accounts of treatment and what treatment enacts.

The Treatment of Endometriosis

Women diagnosed with endometriosis will be faced with a range of treatment options. As I have already noted, no treatment has been found to completely eliminate recurrence (Gao, Outley, Botteman, et al. 2006: 1562). Treatment options are usually described as falling into one of four main categories: surgical, drug, dietary and complementary or alternative therapies. Surgery is both a diagnostic tool (indeed, it remains, at the time of writing, the *main* diagnostic tool) as well as a method of treatment. It is important, as well, to distinguish between the different methods and 'aims' of surgery available. Most surgical interventions for the diagnosis and treatment of endometriosis are achieved through the use of a laparoscope. Developed around the turn of the twentieth century, laparoscopy involves the insertion of a lighted tube through a small incision in or near the navel (Phillips and Motta 2000: 32–3).[8] Although it did not become widely available until the 1970s and 1980s (Evans 2005: 32), laparoscopy was used with increased frequency after the turn of the century and had become the recommended diagnostic technique by 1975 (Chalmers 1975).[9] It is now widely regarded as the 'gold standard' diagnostic test (Sutton and Jones 2004: 17).[10] This is partly because laparoscopy is considered a relatively simple operation. It is also understood to be less traumatic for women because it usually requires less recovery time. As well, it is relatively inexpensive and surgery can be completed comparatively quickly. As well as being the principal means of diagnosis, surgery functions as a form of treatment, with endometrial deposits being burnt off (diathermy) or excised during laparoscopy. Through the laparoscope, the surgeon inspects the pelvic organs and drains fluid, destroys growths, frees adhesions, and removes large endometrial growths (Phillips and Motta 2000: 32–3). In some cases the entire uterus and/ or ovaries will also be removed via hysterectomy (sometimes through keyhole surgery, and sometimes through a more invasive procedure). In many cases the disease recurs after surgery including hysterectomy, which has been found to be the most effective treatment available, in that women who have had the treatment have the lowest rates of recurrence (Winkel 2003 cited in Gao, Outley, Botteman, et al. 2006: 1562).

---

8   Steptoe (1967: 1) claims that Kelling was the first to experiment with the method. Surgery was performed upon a dog and Kelling's results on the use of the technique were published in 1901. The laparoscope was reportedly used for a gynaecological procedure as early as 1912, by Nordentoeft of Denmark (Steptoe 1967: 1).

9   Similarly, just four years later, in the *Handbook of Obstetrics and Gynaecology*, it is recommended, alongside laparotomy, to enable diagnosis (Wren 1979: 405).

10   Despite the fact that laparoscopy is regarded as the most reliable method of diagnosing endometriosis there is some evidence that its use may be reduced in the future. In 2006, the United Kingdom's Royal College of Obstetricians and Gynaecologists (RCOG) released a set of guidelines for the investigation and management of endometriosis and highlighted problems with the use of laparoscopy as a primary diagnostic measure, because of the risk of complications associated with the surgery (RCOG 2006: 3). Women who display symptoms of endometriosis but who have not been diagnosed through laparoscopy might be administered a hormonal treatment to reduce or eliminate menstrual flow whilst her progress is monitored (Kennedy, Bergqvist, Chapron, D'Hooghe, et al. 2005: 2698). Other methods for diagnosis continue to be under investigation.

Drug therapies are another common treatment and range from those aimed at managing pain to those designed to stem the growth of endometrial tissue by suppressing hormonal activity or the entire menstrual cycle for a time (Brewer 1995: 64). The stated aim of most medical treatments is to alter the menstrual cycle to produce what is often described as a state of pseudo-pregnancy or pseudo-menopause (Olive and Pritts 2001: 266). The expectation here is that the state of pseudo-pregnancy/menopause will provide less-than-optimal conditions for the growth of the endometrium, and thus, endometrial implants (Olive and Pritts 2001: 266). One of the most common types of drug treatment offered to women are Gonadotropin-releasing hormone (GnRH) agonists – which impact upon the secretion of both follicle-stimulating hormone (FSL) and luteinising hormone (Olive and Pritts 2001: 267) and purport to reduce the secretion of oestrogen (Makita, Ishitana, Ohta, et al. 2005: 392). The most common method of administering the GnRH agonists is by injection beneath the skin (Kiesel, Rody, Greb, et al. 2002: 679). Administration of GnRH agonists cause hypogonadotropic hypogonadism (Olive and Pritts 2001: 267) or a state of absent or decreased functioning of the ovaries, atrophy of the endometrium and the cessation of the menstrual period (Olive and Pritts 2001: 267). Most patients have tried some combination of the above treatments (Cox et al. 2003b). Drug treatments for pain symptoms are available, commonly including non-steroidal anti-inflammatory drugs – or NSAIDS (Olive and Pritts 2001: 268). Several studies have found that hormonal drug treatments can relieve painful symptoms associated with endometriosis (see Olive and Pritts 2001: 268–9).

Recently there has been an increased emphasis on dietary changes and/or alternative treatments such as acupuncture in order to manage the condition. The range of treatments on offer here is extensive, and reflects the heterogeneity of ideas about the aetiology of endometriosis, as well as possible strategies for its prevention, as I discussed in chapters 1 and 2. As I briefly flagged at the outset of the book, a number of recent studies have positioned endometriosis as a disease of lifestyle. In the medical literature, it has been suggested that there could be a relationship between the condition and diet, exercise, smoking, caffeine, alcohol, chocolate or cannabis (Parazzini, Chiaffarino, Surace, et al. 2004; Missmer and Cramer 2003; Moen 1994). In addition, there are possible links between endometriosis and changes in the environment, especially the utilisation of chemicals such as polychlorinated biphenyls, or PCBs (see Mills and Vernon 2002: 217). As I explained in earlier chapters, especially Chapter 3, possible routes of exposure to xeno-oestrogens, PCBs and dioxins are extensive and treatment regimens often focus on avoiding them. So, as I noted earlier, women with endometriosis may engage in a range of lifestyle and/or dietary changes – including those I mention in chapters 3 and 5 – in order to try and manage the disease.

Although these are the most commonly recognised forms of treatment for women, in practice, women described other treatment regimens, and other injunctions to treatment. Maddy was advised by her herbalist, for instance, to take steps that would minimise the risks and effects of retrograde menstruation:

> [The naturopath said] that when my period is due, or when I have actually got my period, don't lie with my legs above my pelvis. She was very firm in the belief that this could actually make things worse. If my back is hurting or my legs are aching or whatever, then yeah, put your feet up. That's fine. But always keep them tilted at a level that is not – so that they are not raised above my pelvis … It is an unusual one, but I have taken it on board and live by it.

The point here is that women may engage with treatments beyond the few main examples I have described above. The first of two treatment regimens I want to examine is also one not often acknowledged in mainstream biomedical literature, but which many women I interviewed encountered. This involves the suggestion to treat the disease by having a baby.

The Will to Pregnancy

Many women that I interviewed for this study explained that their physicians encouraged them to opt for pregnancy as a way of treating the condition. This advice was offered in spite of the current scientific consensus that pregnancy does not cure the disease (Evans 2005: 14).[11] According to some of the women, moreover, pregnancy was offered as the main form of treatment, or it was privileged over and above other options (such as hormonal treatment). Some women were advised that pregnancy would likely be a cure-all for endometriosis, in that it would, as Mary put it, 'wipe out' their disease. As another participant, Stephanie, explained:

> With the gynaecologist, she was very into trying to get me pregnant. That was her idea of, I guess, curing everything for me. And she really wanted me to just get pregnant and that was all she was recommending as a treatment … It was a bit hard to deal with at 25. I didn't even think of that kind of thing. I wasn't married, I had no idea whether I would stay with my partner. I [did] get married to him eventually, [but at that stage] to get pregnant with him didn't sound right. I thought this was crazy, you can't keep telling me to do this.

Later in the interview, Stephanie explained how the emphasis on fertility:

---

11   Although I do not wish to deny the significance of this as a political and ethical issue, my concern in this chapter is less with the ethics of potentially 'inaccurate' advice being delivered to patients in the clinic, then it is with the various ways in which an injunction such as this may work in the broader sense that Barad (2007, 2003) or even Butler (1993, 1990) would suggest.

frustrated me, it scared me, it, we were actually planning an overseas trip at the time and it just, I didn't know what to do. I was sort of really frustrated by the whole process and quite fed up with it.

Like Stephanie, other interviewees were discouraged by what they perceived as biomedicine's preoccupation with pregnancy. Penelope, for example, was sceptical about the prospect that pregnancy might cure endometriosis and described it as a likely 'urban myth'. Despite her cynicism regarding the biomedical emphasis upon reproduction, however, she became concerned about her fertility after her doctors repeatedly advised her to have children. As she explained:

I get told – especially since I've probably been the age of 21 – that pregnancy would be a very good option for me and it – that thought process – happens regularly. I'm 28, my D-day is actually 30, apparently … it's still something that is in my brain and that looms.

Read together, the accounts of Stephanie and Penelope offer important insights into the way that medicine materialises subjecthood. Both accounts of the clinical encounter suggest two vital assumptions underpinning the biomedical approach to the disease. It is assumed, first, that women *want* to have children, and secondly, that they *can* have them. Both assumptions perform a version of agency that is, I argue, crucial to the particular version of subjecthood that treatment makes available to women. More specifically, both accounts perform the ability to have a child (as well as the absence of one) as an exercise of free will. These versions of agency resonate with most medical accounts of that phenomenon, discussed earlier in this book, of 'delayed' parenthood. In such medical accounts, the deferral of parenthood is almost always exclusively attributed to women and portrayed as a product of women's 'agency'. Partners (if they exist) almost never figure as playing a role in the achievement of pregnancy, nor as having any responsibility in the decision to have a child. Because of the assumptions that appear to flow through clinical encounters about treatment, and because of the particular version of agency that is embodied therein, women who later fail to produce a child are immediately conferred with a particular, politically potent status: that of the 'delaying' mother.

This subject position materialises through a dynamic process of material-discursive intra-action: where injunctions to treat endometriosis through pregnancy coalesce with women's biological status as 'non-pregnant' and/or 'non-parous'. This subject position does not pre-date the clinical encounter, but, crucially, emerges within it, as assumptions about women's reproductive desires and physical capacities are applied, injunctions to pregnancy are made, and pregnancy, finally, is not realised. Crucially, pregnancy was not in consideration for either Penelope or Stephanie prior to the clinical encounter, and insofar as it was not of interest or concern to them, neither was the possibility that they were exercising their agency to 'delay' or 'defer' anything at all. The 'delaying' mother is thus a product of the clinic itself, a hugely significant event for the politics of the disease, not in the least because it is a highly politicised and ethically charged one. Most obviously, every time a woman is performed as 'deferring' reproduction, she is simultaneously performed as culpable insofar as pregnancy is simultaneously enacted as a useful means for curing one's own illness.

Women who occupy the devalued subject position that I have described here have only one way of etching out a less stigmatised subject position: by producing a child. For the reasons I have already outlined, however, some of which include women's physical inability to bear children, this is not always achievable. According to the women that I interviewed, the role of infertility is rarely raised in those clinical settings where pregnancy is recommended. The failure of medical discourses to engage with the possibility that infertility will impact women's ability to treat the disease through pregnancy – even if pregnancy might have an effect – is nothing short of extraordinary, given that infertility is understood as one of the main symptoms of endometriosis. Doctors appear to be recommending a form of treatment that for a large number of women is likely to be unavailable. And to the extent that infertility is often distressing and a source of stigma in and of itself (Riessman 2002), it is deeply concerning that physicians might not engage with these complexities as and when they propose pregnancy as a treatment.

Individual women who do produce children may find themselves transformed into a new kind of subject: one that has exercised her agency 'appropriately'. Indeed, countless newspaper reports about the horrors of living with the disease often conclude with the 'triumph' of childbirth, as if to suggest that the arrival of a child signals the end of suffering. Triumphant narratives such as these also operate as a potent reminder to all women with endometriosis that they have failed, both as subjects and citizens, if they do not produce children. In a personal and political sense, these configurations have major implications for women with endometriosis, especially those women who do not have children, regardless of the reasons why. As well as this, as I will explain, the production of 'delayed' motherhood also raises questions about the epidemic more broadly.

The Demands of Time

Time features in all women's accounts of the injunction to pregnancy, as well, of course, in the notion of 'delayed' motherhood. Penelope, we will recall, had been encouraged to fall pregnant since at least the age of 21. As well as developing a heightened sensitivity about the need to have a baby (a thought process that she said now 'happens regularly'), she also had a timeline in mind: 'I'm 28, my D-day is actually 30, apparently … it's still something that is in my brain and that looms.' Time figures centrally, as well, in Miriam's account of the injunction to pregnancy:

[My gynaecologist] knew I was single at that time. He said: "If your social circumstances permit you, if you are going to have children, then I would recommend that you would get on with it by the time you are 35." And I am going "Shit, OK I am 34, or just 33 going on 34". So I had my 34th birthday thinking "Hmm, not a man in sight". So suddenly having children seemed to be the most important thing and who gives a stuff about career. I don't care. So I was so miserable. It was something I always thought, "Oh I might maybe one day", but I felt like I had several years of good child breeding in me if I should meet the right person. But suddenly that [length of time] was contracted.

Although Chelsea was not initially concerned with her fertility, she became worried through her consultations with doctors. She came to understand endometriosis as being about more than pain (her main symptom) and as 'a whole package of things that had to be dealt with', the most important of which, according to her physician, was fertility. Endometriosis was reconfigured as a reproductive disorder. With this, Chelsea's 'orientation' to life – and crucially, to time – changed:

Suddenly, you know, you have got to think just about what is going on with your body now, what is going to go on with your body in the future, always quite preoccupied, it takes up a lot of my mental space, for a long time thinking about how is this story going to play out.

Like Miriam, the injunction to pregnancy to which Chelsea was subject was bounded in time, as her doctor:

put a lot of pressure on me around fertility issues, which really just freaked me out because it was something that I had never thought of. I was 18, it was not anything I wanted to think about and suddenly there was someone going "well you need to think about these things, you need to have children by 28". Suddenly all these issues that had never really occurred to me before. So I guess it came, it was not just about learning I was sick, it was like a whole different lifestyle and a whole package of things that had to be dealt with.

Both Miriam and Chelsea's accounts mobilise and reproduce time as a key factor in the need to reproduce. It is their understanding – in part through the way their doctors delivered these injunctions – that the best chances of pregnancy having an ameliorative effect on the disease lie in the achievement of pregnancy in *good time*.

In this way, both accounts perform a set of normative temporal relations. What I mean by this is that both accounts reflect and reproduce a version of time as linear, but also – crucially – as linked to the maintenance of order. Enfolded within the notion of delayed parenthood are at least two important assumptions that bear upon time: first, that life events are *supposed* to progress in a particular way and in a specific order, on the one hand, and second, that one of the features of *ordered time* is achievement of parenthood. Injunctions to treat endometriosis through pregnancy therefore rely on a version of time as linear, and reinforce the central features of normative and ordered life. Because delayed parenthood is linked so closely to the development and progression of the disease, endometriosis has to be understood, symbolically-literally and materially as an 'effect' of disordered time. Together these movements render women's failure to reproduce 'in time' (for whatever reason) as a form of disorder. One of the effects of this is that the will to pregnancy is rendered as a demand – not of medicine 'itself', but of time. In this way, accounts of the will to pregnancy function to assign agency in two senses: first, to women, as I have already outlined, and then, to time, which figures as having its own expectations of women, independent of both medicine and the 'social'.

Hormonal Therapies

The other form of treatment that I want to examine in this chapter is hormonal drug therapy. As I have already noted, there are a diverse range of hormonal therapies available for women. It is generally recognised that treatments can bring severe side effects including weight gain, lethargy, mood changes, depression, nausea, hot flushes, sweats, oily skin, changes to appetite, decreased libido, muscular pain, vaginal dryness, headaches, thinning of the bones, insomnia, irreversible deepening of the voice, irreversible liver damage, increased hair growth, abnormal bleeding, breast tenderness and fluid retention (Evans 2005: 63–8; Olive and Pritts 2001: 266). In recent years, physicians have sought to minimise these side effects through the administration of hormonal add-back therapy similar to the kind often prescribed to menopausal women (Makita, Ishitana, Ohta, et al. 2005; Surrey and Hornstein 2002; Olive and Pritts 2001: 268; Hornstein, Surrey, Weisberg, et al. 1998). Most of the women I interviewed had tried hormonal therapies of some kind or another – sometimes with add-back therapy – and in most instances, understood themselves to have experienced at least some of these reported side effects. In the following excerpt, Mary explains her understanding of the nature and purpose of hormonal therapy, along with her experiences of it:

> Basically as it was explained to me – and I mean I haven't looked up any of this information so I may have misunderstood it or misread it or whatever – at the time but this is the way that I see it. It was basically a male hormone and it put your body into like a, to give you the idea, put in certain hormones to raise your testosterone level, your oestrogen levels are therefore less in the body and that happens when you are pregnant and when you go through a pregnancy the hormones usually get rid of the endometriosis. But the theory behind having this medication was it was trying to change the levels of testosterone in the body to let the body, you know, to help fight this thing. I went on it for 9 months and in the 9 month period, I lost the plot completely and my father would even probably tell you, I just turned feral, I would even pick fights in the pub. I'm 5

foot 2 inches, at the time I probably weighed about 45 kilos, you know, and I'm not an angry person, and I'm not a drunk, you know what I mean I was just that aggressive and umm [the] hair growth was terrible. Aches as well, I got from it, so that's 9 months I was on this treatment and I hated it … After that stuff that I had, look you know I remember punching my dad. I punched my brother. Look, it was just awful. I cried all the time, and I didn't know what was wrong with me, and I was up and down and moody. Yeah it was just not right at all.

Here, Mary understands herself to have been *transformed* into a new kind of subject by the medication she has taken – to have become someone else entirely: someone who is more aggressive, moody, hairy and emotional. There are several things that can be said about this. First, Mary constructs the medication as masculinising in its materiality and its effects, describing the particular drug that she took as a 'male' hormone. Here, Mary is enacting a version of hormonal medication in which the drug is imbued with a set of pre-existing attributes and qualities. The hormone is responsible for producing a set of changes in her physical and emotional state, seemingly an unintended consequence of the drug's disruption of the 'natural' balance of hormones in her body.

In these ways, Mary's account of endometriosis treatment enacts a particular, normative version of hormones and the way that they operate upon men and women, where hormones are understood to be the cause of physical and emotional alterations. Mary's account shares much with conventional understandings of hormones as either the bodily 'messengers' of sex (Roberts 2007), or the 'essence' of sexual difference (Oudshoorn 1994). In this sense, Mary both produces and reproduces the idea that hormones possess inherent properties and that they act upon the natural body in ways that are either inherently stabilising or destabilising. To some extent, there are overlaps with the way that she sees herself whilst on medication and the way that women in the next chapter describe themselves with endometriosis, as we shall see: as inauthentic, unstable, irrational and monstrous. Here, however, Mary actively attributes these aspects of her behaviour to the drug (and to hormones). In this way, she assigns agency and responsibility for her 'feral' mood and problematic subjectivity to something external to her '*self*'. This designation departs in important ways from the way that the women with endometriosis sometimes assign responsibility for the 'problematic' behaviour they understand themselves to be exhibiting – a concept I take up in more detail in the next chapter. At the same time, Mary's account of treatment folds back upon conventional understandings of drugs and hormones as chaotic within this particular context, in their materiality and their effects. This also represents a departure from conventional understandings of medical treatment as inherently stabilising and as productive of order (although see Illich, 1976, for example, for a contrary view).

Other women had a similar understanding of their treatment, although some demonstrated a more complicated view of the way the treatment regime functioned. As Chelsea explained, for instance:

> [My medication] is called Zoladex … I'm like most people. I have found it really good. It had given me my entire quality of life back. I got to the point before where I was saying to my doctor and my gynaecologist you can't let me have another period. I can't walk with it. I can't do anything. I just feel so much pain. You just can't let me, I won't do it anymore … So I think for a lot of people who would probably go on this treatment, it would seem like the side effects are pretty horrible, I mean just the menopause side effects … I think now I have been on it for so long, and haven't had periods for 7 years, I do get funny about it, I don't feel particularly womanly when you are essentially menopausal at the age of 20, and there are a lot of issues around that that bother me because of the treatment. But I certainly like it better than any other contraceptive pills which never helped me one damn bit.

In this excerpt, Chelsea expresses a more complicated and perhaps even ambivalent relationship to her treatment than Mary. On the one hand, Zoladex has given Chelsea her 'quality of life back', with her pain becoming more manageable. On the other hand, she feels that the treatment has made her less 'womanly'. Like Mary, Chelsea enacts drug treatment as an inherently masculinising process and reproduces conventional understandings of 'nature', 'gender' and what hormones 'do'. Both women understand hormonal therapy to have acted upon them in such a way that they now exceed the boundaries of acceptable and normative femininity. For both Mary and Chelsea, the failure to menstruate and the expression of aggression are signifiers of the 'masculine'. Although these might be valorised among men, they don't accord with normative femininity. In this sense, treatment works to perform both women in ways that they recognise and enact as disavowed.

Chelsea's experiences might be contrasted to those of another woman, Miriam, who understood the treatment to have produced a range of very debilitating effects. As she explained in this lengthy excerpt:

> And so it must have been like 3 weeks or some more into taking the Zoladex, suddenly I went ah, hot flush. It wasn't like I was sweating, I never got sweat thank god, but yeah I started noticing symptoms … certainly going onto the Zoladex helped [the menstrual] pain. And basically I got to this point of being pain free. I felt I was sliding gradually into this more, you know, hugely anxious depressed state … I thought I was just down in the dumps because, I was down in the dumps, and I had been down in the dumps for a very long time, but I haven't sort of twigged that, I had forgotten, I don't know, that depression is a side effect of menopausal symptoms. So I was gradually deteriorating and it got to the point where I was finding it very hard to make small decisions and everything seemed really stressful. [Eventually] I went to pieces in front of my boss. I said I was depressed, I wasn't coping. I felt like I had two heads. I had never felt so desperate, this is the depression, the hormonal depression. I just felt this sheer desperation, and people were saying well desperation *for what*? I couldn't tell you, just desperation. I was ringing psychiatric triage lines and all

of this sort of stuff and I'm thinking I need a psychiatrist because I'm just like, you know, it's a hormonal thing. I am just going crazy, I felt like I was going mad. And I saw [the doctor] again for another periodic check-up and I had said I am so not coping, I think. And [the doctor] said what has been going on the last few weeks, and he is like umm well it could very well be the Zoladex.

Unlike Chelsea, Miriam emphasises the emotional 'effects' of Zoladex, and a range of psychological symptoms that she experienced whilst on the drug. In attributing these symptoms to the drug, Miriam performs Zoladex as inherently psychologically destabilising and debilitating. Importantly, however, she also emerges through treatment as the kind of subject that has so often been associated with the disease: overly emotional, irrational, overanxious, and so on. Even though the career woman's designator has been thoroughly critiqued in recent years, it is impossible to ignore the parallels between the account that Miriam gives of herself in treatment and the one so often offered in portrayals of the 'typical' endometriotic subject. Like Mary, there are also overlaps with the idea of the 'monstrous feminine' that I will discuss more fully in the next chapter, in the sense that Miriam understands her emotional state to be inherently problematic and shameful. Several women I interviewed reported experiences similar to the ones that Miriam so graphically describes here. In Internet chat forums, self-help literature, media reports and blogs, similar accounts of treatment can be found, and many women – including some I interviewed for this study, experience suicidal ideations that they attribute to their medication. In an earlier study I conducted, one interviewee vividly detailed how, after commencing treatment, she became so depressed that she fantasised about slamming her head through plate glass so as to end her mental anguish (Seear 2004).

Accounts such as these raise serious questions about the efficacy and ethics of administering hormonal treatment to some women. Perhaps in recognition of this, physicians are currently subject to restrictions in the use of some hormonal therapies for women with the disease. There are limitations on the length of time that women can be allowed to stay on certain drugs, for example, because of concerns about the possible side effects associated with long-term use. So, as Juanita explained:

I remember when Zoladex came on the market, you could only have it for 6 months in your life. These things are super heavy duty. There is a whole lot of male gunk in there, which you are putting in your body to try and readjust your own feminine hormones, and chemistry. That's heavy-duty stuff. That sort of caveat was put on it because they didn't know what the effects of it were going to be long term.

In this example, Juanita performs Zoladex as being replete with 'male gunk', and, like Mary and Chelsea, inherently masculinising in its effects. Importantly, she also understands it to operate upon one's existing 'chemistry'. This accords with Celia

Roberts' (2007: 194) approach to hormones. As Roberts has previously explained, hormones are usually understood to have a 'disciplining' function insofar as they can be utilised to restore order and balance to deviant bodies through re-establishing acceptable boundaries between the sexes, as in the case, for instance, of men experiencing erectile dysfunction. In that instance, the ability to generate and maintain an erection is understood as a key signifier of masculinity and of sex difference. Hormonal therapies like the popular drug Viagra are understood to enable the *restoration* of normative masculinity. In this sense, then, Viagra operates to both maintain and reinforce understandings of what masculinity 'is', and – importantly – what it is not. Viagra thus produces the flaccid penis, in Butler's terms, as symbolically connected to the 'domain of the abject'. As this example and the accounts of Juanita, Mary and Chelsea remind us, hormones have assumed a central sociocultural function in contemporary society, operating to produce both the subject and the abject. Even when hormones are understood to disrupt 'natural' bodies and the established order in ways that are potentially negative (through producing women that are too aggressive, for instance), hormones are working to maintain and reproduce these normative boundaries. In a way, women understand hormones to be centrally implicated in the production of the woman-as-cyborg, a figure I examined briefly in Chapter 1. Hormones are intimately connected with the production of a very particular and politically potent version of disordered femininity. Significantly, of course, breaching the boundaries of normative femininity is understood to be implicated in the development of the disease and the epidemic – a subject I will return to towards the end of this chapter.

Treatment and Non-compliance

In both of the treatment contexts I have examined here, women emerge as *non-compliant* patients who have failed to adhere to medical advice. As I have discussed elsewhere (Seear 2009d), compliance with medical advice is almost always valorised as a hallmark of responsible citizenship in late modern, Western discursive contexts. This is yet another example of the political and ethical function of medical treatment. Some forms of treatment, that is, produce some women as disavowed subjects: every failure to comply with pregnancy advice produces women, by extension, as non-compliant. Sometimes this works through women's active rejection of medical advice. Although three of the women in the study – Wanda, Chelsea and Barbara – had been advised to consider treating endometriosis through pregnancy whilst they were in their late teens, none complied with that treatment direction. According to all three, this advice was offered despite the fact that they had not expressed any desire for children in the clinical encounter and despite none of them having a partner with whom they wished to have children (even though this is not, of course, a necessity). Barbara felt that the prospect of her giving birth at such a young age, without a partner to support her and whilst suffering from a debilitating medical condition was absurd: 'who's going to raise the child?' Here, Barbara appraises the injunction to pregnancy using her own (embodied) logic, but this kind of rationale is not always well received by treating doctors. One of the women, Hannah, felt that her treating doctors focussed almost entirely upon injunctions to pregnancy and that she was criticised as a result:

> I guess every time I go to the doctors, they just keep bringing up about having kids, "[you have] got to have kids, got to get rid of it, got to have kids" and I'm getting a little bit sick of that argument, because I ended up at the last visit saying "Well, I am not ready to have kids" ... I said I'm not having them if I'm not ready ... It's not like we are here to discuss this, it's the "you should be, you are doing yourself damage by not considering this option" you know?

In this excerpt, Hannah emerges as a non-compliant patient, via her refusal to bear children. There is also a direct and palpable sense within which she is constructed as responsible for her own predicament. It is not entirely clear what 'damage' is supposed to mean within this context. It may be a reference to disease progression in general, or to the possible effects of disease progression on Hannah's fertility, or both. Either way, Hannah comes away from the clinical encounter with a sense of herself as potentially culpable, and as deviant. This is an invariably stigmatising space to occupy.

Similar examples were found in my interviews with women about their uptake – or more precisely, their *refusal* to uptake – hormonal therapies. A small number of women decided against hormonal treatment, either because of their own experiences with medication, or through second-hand accounts of the side effects experienced by other women. Stephanie, for example, came across accounts of the side effects of treatment on the Internet, and decided that hormonal therapy was not something she wanted to explore:

> I guess I [was] just reading into what the hormones could do and all of the side-effects and the fact that in some instances, although it was quite rare, in some instances the side-effects couldn't be reversed once you got off the medication. And again I was just reading a lot of different online chat groups and things like that and the many women who were talking about the medications that they were on and there were more negative stories than positive ones. I just didn't want to put myself in that situation.

The decision to reject medical treatment is not an easy one for these women. The complexity of these decisions was articulated best by Miriam, who was cognisant that:

> the risks were, you know, I could be losing bone density and end up, I thought, oh my god, am I going to end up with an old woman's body, osteoporosis, and all that? So I felt between a rock and a hard place, like there was nowhere to turn.

Hormonal therapies taken by women with endometriosis are not uncontroversial. Some drugs have been – or presently are – the subject of lawsuits in countries including the United States, in part because women claim to have experienced very severe adverse reactions to them.[12] At the very least, then, we must wonder why it is that women's refusal to engage with these treatments might ever be positioned as an instance of problematic non-compliance and a marker of irresponsible citizenship. Daisy started hormonal therapy and explained that:

> I stayed on [the hormone treatment] continuously so I wouldn't menstruate, and it didn't agree with me at all, at all. My face, my body, and everything just swelled up. I got really puffy, and was putting on a lot of weight and from looking at pictures of me and I thought oh my goodness, and could see that there was something wrong, the hormones were not agreeing with me, and the pain got much worse, yeah, much worse ... I was just getting sicker and sicker through it all. [After a while] I thought to myself I am not putting myself through this, it is obvious the hormone treatment was not working ... You know, I didn't feel [my doctors] were honest with me about the side effects. And when I told them the side effects I was having, they were very reluctant to relate it to the drug. They would say "what am I eating", or "how am I sleeping?" Just, I don't know, with some of the drugs they had on the market, [I wondered] how much research they had done on them, with the particular one I was on.

In this example, Daisy understood her doctors to doubt the cause of her symptoms, and, as such, to doubt *her*. Of course it is entirely possible that neither she nor her doctors are right, or that both are right, or that something else is at work here. The key point, however, is that Daisy's understanding of her own symptoms and the origin of those symptoms – an account which accords with most medical literature on the effects of hormonal therapy – seems to have been discounted. Instead, as I have already argued, Daisy's practitioners recast her as a difficult and insufficiently obedient patient. In this way, Daisy deviates from the expectations associated with Western, liberal discursive subjecthood, as well as the normative feminine role, where she is expected to be more passive, respectful of authority, and to uncritically accept the views of those experts who are treating her. In her own account, Daisy is constituted as the very kind of 'typical' endometriotic subject – headstrong, intelligent, resistant, and overcomplicated – that is presumed to pre-exist her treatment. This raises questions about the role that treatment plays in the constitution of the epidemic 'itself'.

---

12   I am indebted to Celia Roberts for bringing to my attention some of the controversies surrounding Lupron, for example.

Treatment, Typical Patients and the Epidemic

Among other things, the analysis I have undertaken in this chapter should raise questions about the way that cause and effect are understood within the context of epidemics. As I have noted already, the materialisation of endometriosis as an epidemic has several claimed associations and origins. One common explanation for the emergence of the epidemic relates to the attributes, traits, 'behaviour' or agency of women with the condition; all of which, as I have already explained, are said to pre-date women's enrolment in treatment. According to this approach, nulliparous women are at risk of developing the disease through, as Kennedy (2005) reminds us, increased 'exposure' to menstruation. Increased exposure, as I also discussed in Chapter 2, is frequently mobilised as likely to be implicated in the disease, with the decision to defer pregnancy being critical in at least two ways: first, to the development of the disease, and later, for women who have already been diagnosed with the condition, to its progression. In this sense it is often claimed that late, modern western societies are increasingly characterised by women's failure to reproduce – or at least their deferral of motherhood, and that these changes in thinking and behaviour are centrally implicated in a spike in disease incidence. Similarly, as I have already noted, accounts of endometriosis frequently presume that women possess certain inherent character traits and that these are precursors for disease development, as well as the epidemic.

As I have argued throughout this chapter, however, the 'typical' patients that are apparently both prior to and implicated in the making of the epidemic are actually *made in treatment*. Treatment therefore plays a central role – not just in the production of subjecthood – but also in the production of the disease/epidemic itself. This is a largely circular process whereby medical knowledge and practice folds back upon itself. So, as I explained at the outset of this chapter, endometriosis medicine assumes one of its roles to be the identification and management of pre-existing subject types. Doctors look for certain types of women, believing them to be predisposed to the disease. In treatment, assumptions are also made about the characteristics of the women being treated, and about the relationships between this and disease progression, prevention, prognosis, and so forth. In a reversal of this realist logic, however, I want to suggest that the identification, isolation and materialisation of these 'typical patients' is generated *via* these pre-existing ideas and assumptions. In this way, treatment co-constitutes the very kinds of subjects it purports to treat, subjects that are central, as I have suggested, to understandings of 'cause' and 'effect' in the making of the modern epidemic. Following on from this, medicine strengthens its own claims that the number of 'typical patients' is on the rise, and that the disease-epidemic is on the rise as a 'consequence' of this. This is a perfect example of the point I made earlier in the book, following Judith Butler (1990: 37), that the processes by which subjects and objects are made are 'effectively concealed', or forgotten, amidst all of this activity. The materiality of the epidemic – which includes disease incidence and prevalence, but also other symptoms of disease, such as disease progression – is actually better understood as a phenomenon that emerges through treatment. What this means, then, is that the endometriosis epidemic is both a thoroughly biomedical object, and a sociocultural phenomenon. As a multifarious phenomenon, endometriosis is shaped and formed, literally and metaphorically, through complex means. This calls for new ways of thinking through disease management and treatment, including, crucially, more critical thinking about the role medicine plays in producing the very 'problems' it seeks to address.

Conclusion

In this chapter I have argued that medical treatment for women with endometriosis has a central function in the constitution of subjects. Importantly, just as there is more than one form of treatment available for women with endometriosis (and, moreover, women may take up some, none, or a combination of available therapies), more than one subject position is constituted in practice. Indeed, with several kinds of treatment available, *treatment intra-actively constitutes a range of subject positions*. It is tempting to conclude that the number of subject positions made available through treatment is as broad and deep as the range of treatments themselves. The danger here is in enacting a kind of pluralism of the kind that has already been the subject of extensive critique (e.g. Mol 2002). I suggest that it is more useful to describe endometriosis treatment as producing more than one kind of subject, but less than many, following Mol (2002). The subjects produced in treatment align very clearly with the 'typical patient profile' – variously manifested over the years – that figures centrally in endometriosis discourse. Accordingly, endometriosis treatment produces the very subjects it claims to be treating. As well as this, to the extent that subjectivity is understood as *causal* in the production and distribution of the disease, treatment must also be understood as having a central role in the materialisation of the epidemic. In understanding the epidemic as an intra-actively co-constituted phenomenon, I do not mean to question the 'reality' of the disease or its incidence, nor to suggest that matter is 'passive and immutable' (Barad 2003: 801) so that the disease is a kind of fiction. Instead, the point is that epidemics *are more than merely biological (or, for that matter, discursive) phenomena*: they are co-constituted through a range of practices and processes, including processes that are understood to be largely (or even exclusively) the realm of 'the social', or of 'culture'. Thinking about the endometriosis epidemic in this way is, I suggest, a positive development, because it lends to new ways of thinking about the making of the disease and new ways for tackling it, including ways that go beyond the 'merely' biological or biomedical.

I want to conclude this chapter with some thoughts about the ethics and politics of treatment, and ways that the administration of treatment might be reconsidered. Starting with the question of pregnancy, I suggest that physicians need to reconsider the way they approach clinical encounters. For the reasons I have already explained, it is vital that physicians re-appraise their own assumptions about women, including the assumption that most (if not all) women will desire to have children. Women with endometriosis are a diverse population, and although some will desire children, some will not. Importantly, assumptions about women's capacities to reproduce need to be avoided, wherever possible, as this only works to perform reproduction as a matter of women's agency – a problematic phenomenon that may provoke self-blame among those women who want to have children, but are unfortunately unable to. In all of these ways, the problem seems to partially derive from the fact that clinical interactions are less patient-centered or patient-directed than they could be. According to the women I interviewed, it is the *physicians* that drive the priorities and parameters established within the clinical interaction. Although some women will prefer it this way, one of the effects of this may be to privilege the physician's own assumptions about what women will want to know, be concerned about, etc., so that fertility issues may be positioned as more important than women's primary concerns, such as pain. Although it is always possible that a physician will still end up recommending pregnancy as a cure for pain, it is also possible that the assumptions about women's desires and capacities informs treatment recommendations, so that all of these things are conflated within the context of the clinic. A more careful and considered discussion of all of these issues, along with alternatives to pregnancy, such as in-vitro fertilisation and adoption, should women desire this information, could also do much to lessen the stigma association with non-parity.

On the other hand, as I have already explained, drug therapies for the disease remain controversial and raise a number of questions about the ethics of biomedicine. There is no doubt that many women understand hormonal therapies as beneficial for them, as the accounts in this chapter show. But we also need to acknowledge that many women do not experience these therapies as beneficial, or that some experience a combination of what they understand to be positive and negative effects. My research shows that physicians may not always be attuned to the diversity of women's experiences, including, for example, the possibility that treatment generates considerable emotional distress. It is especially concerning that in spite of medical literature reporting these side effects, and women's regular accounts of same, some women's treating physicians continue to doubt the veracity of women's claims, so that they attribute these problems to women themselves. At the very least there may be a need for improved medical education in this respect, as many physicians openly acknowledge. I have attended many forums, conferences and meetings in which gynaecologists and other specialists openly acknowledge the confusion and limited understanding of the disease within the medical profession as a whole, and the tendency for some doctors to perpetuate harmful stereotypes about women through trivialising their symptoms and concerns. There have been attempts to address this for a long time including, for example, through the annual worldwide Endometriosis Awareness Day, which aims to engage both women and experts in a greater dialogue around the disease, and to raise public awareness about the seriousness of it. Awareness Days afford one – albeit limited – opportunity to address these issues, but there are many other spaces where these misunderstandings could be addressed. These include, for example, medical education at both undergraduate and postgraduate levels, medical literature and continuing professional development, especially for general practitioners, whose understanding of the disease and new treatments may be limited.

Finally, I hope that questions might begin to be asked about the 'benefits' and 'effects' of treatment more broadly. As my analysis indicates, treatment sometimes generates stigma and shame, and has the potential, in confluence with other factors, to render women as culpable for aspects of their ill-health. This is an extremely worrying phenomenon, and one that is almost always overlooked in discussions about endometriosis treatment – even those that suggest treatment might be harmful to women. The potential for medicine to produce harms has long been understood. Unfortunately, however, there is a tendency to conceptualise medical harms in a narrow way, framed by biomedical and scientific understandings of 'harm', but also 'cause' and 'effect'. If we accept that medical treatment sometimes performs women with endometriosis as grossly dysfunctional, disordered and chaotic subjects, are we not obliged to ask whether treatment of this kind is justified or justifiable? On what basis might it be justified? Is there sufficient research into women's experiences with treatment, and are women given the opportunity to consider all of the information before treatment is offered? How might we reconsider medical treatment, when that treatment has the potential to contribute to the stigmatisation of an already grossly stigmatised population of women (as I would suggest women with endometriosis are)? At the very least I think we need to listen more closely to women's narratives about how treatment was for them – including, but not limited to, their experienced with specific drugs. Mine is one of the few studies in the world to explore these aspects of treatment, but this research has its limitations, and there is a need for more work to be done. Unfortunately, my analysis tends to collapse different drugs together for example, in ways that neglect the specific and localised dimensions of those treatments. I hope more work will be done on this in the future, and that this will generate new ideas about how to approach treatment moving forward. This work is urgent, and is likely to be needed, I suggest, for as long as a cure remains elusive.

Chapter 5
Sooks, Slobs and Monsters: On Responsibility, Self-care and Living with Endometriosis

Woman is literally a monster.

(Aristotle, in Ussher 2006: 1)

I am just an evil monster a few days a month.

(Maddy)

The experience of living with endometriosis is a subject that has been almost entirely overlooked in the social sciences. Most of the extant social scientific literature focuses on women's pre-diagnostic experiences, including, in particular, issues around the delay to diagnosis. Although the diagnostic delay is undoubtedly an important topic,[1] it seems just as vital to consider what happens to women after they finally achieve a diagnosis. One of the most consistent findings to emerge from earlier research is that women engage in practices of 'self-care' – a nebulous and indeterminate concept (at least in its application to endometriosis) which suggests that women become generally more pro-active, assertive and 'responsibilised' in relation to their disease. In previous academic literature, it is often suggested that women take greater responsibility for their disease after diagnosis, experimenting with complementary and alternative medicine, changes to their diets and lifestyle (Ballweg 2003f; Cox, Henderson, Anderson, et al. 2003b; Cox, Henderson, Wood, et al. 2003c). Beyond general references to these practices, however, we know very little about the self-care phenomenon. What, exactly, does 'self-care' involve? If women become more proactive, assertive and 'responsibilised' after diagnosis, what does this entail? How do they manage their health and the disease? What is the significance, if any, of the disease being both incurable and of uncertain aetiology? How do women navigate the plethora of theories about the disease and the injunctions to which they are subjected? And how, perhaps most importantly, do they interpret and explain their practices? This chapter explores the

---

1 Although I acknowledge the considerable difficulties that some women face in having their complaints of pain taken seriously, and the psychological trauma that many women attribute to their treatment in biomedicine, questions around the experience of pain and the diagnostic delay are not my focus here. (I have examined these issues in a separate paper: Seear 2009c.)

phenomenon of self-care, including how it surfaces in women's illness narratives, what it involves and how it functions.

As we will see, there are several reasons why it is important to study self-care among women with endometriosis. As we know from the previous chapters, for instance, women with endometriosis are regularly enjoined to take greater 'control' of their health and disease following diagnosis. The injunctions to which women are subject are diverse, complex and sometimes contradictory. Those injunctions can be difficult to navigate and practically complex to manage. Crucially, such injunctions are deployed within a complex ethical and political landscape for women living with the disease. This is because, as we already know, women have historically had a largely difficult relationship with biomedicine. Medicine has tended to position women as close to nature, passive, weak and irrational, with medicalisation being justified, to a large extent, on claims about women's inherently diseased nature. Endometriosis medicine is in many ways an exemplar of this: within the field, menstruation has been constituted as intrinsically pathological and women with the disease as fundamentally dysfunctional. Although the ways that women act upon and within biomedicine remains the subject of on-going and vigorous debate, there can be no doubt that medicine – especially gynaecological medicine – has handled women and men unevenly, with a range of deleterious effects. As such, the apparent 'turn' to self-care may signal a shift in the way medicine operates with respect to women and gender, as women move away from mainstream medicine and explore new and alternative methods of care. As a potentially politically and ethically significant process, then, self-care demands urgent attention and careful analysis. What does self-care involve? How does it emerge? How do women interpret their actions? What does self-care mean for gender, agency and power? In what follows, I consider, first, some of the claims made in academic literature regarding the nature of women's self-care and the benefits associated with women taking greater responsibility for their health. I deal then with the broader theoretical literature on these issues, including literature exploring the interrelationship between medical power, responsibility, freedom and agency. Finally, I turn to an analysis of women's narrative accounts of the disease and explore how self-care figures and functions in their lives. I conclude with a consideration of what this all means for medicine, power and gender.

Women, Endometriosis and 'Taking Charge'

In previous studies on how women live with endometriosis, the concepts of responsibility and self-care feature prominently. Women, it is reported, become generally more proactive and responsible following diagnosis, a phenomenon that is seen as largely positive. In one previous study, we are told the story of a woman who experimented with dietary changes and spiritual healing in order to get off 'the medical roundabout' (Cox, Henderson, Anderson, et al. 2003b: 7). In another paper, Cox, Henderson, Wood, et al. (2003c: 66) suggest that women experiment with complementary and alternative medicines in order 'to manage symptoms and obtain some quality of life'. In that study it was said:

> [Women's] dissatisfaction with orthodox medicine was so strong that it resulted in total rejection. There are a variety of reasons for this rejection, ranging from the women having grown tired of the constant need to convince doctors of the legitimacy of their disease and symptoms to wariness of the dangers of repeated invasive treatments, and recognition of the inability of medicine to remove the disease and alleviate its symptoms. (Cox, Henderson, Wood, et al. 2003c: 67)

In the same study, the authors describe this process as one in which women:

> "wrote their own stories" and took charge. This has meant a movement from the margins to the centre, from a position of being powerless to one of being powerful, from being oppressed to being empowered. (Cox, Henderson, Wood, et al. 2003c: 67)

Unfortunately, the claim that women become more 'powerful' as they 'take charge' is not substantiated by any quotes from women themselves. Later in the same study, the authors suggested that:

> Women who had become assertive and taken control of their illness experience argued that they had developed a positive, healing mindset ... These empowered women had discovered that they could live with endometriosis rather than be controlled by it; they remained active rather than withdrawing, and they defined themselves as women who happen to have endometriosis rather than being defined by endometriosis. (Cox, Henderson, Wood, et al. 2003c: 67)

The authors described the process of women taking charge as 'encouraging' (Cox, Henderson, Wood, et al. 2003c: 67). In another study, Cox, Henderson, Anderson, et al. (2003b: 7) claimed that women had taken more control over their lives following diagnosis, and that: 'The women expressed that realising they were ultimately in charge was liberating.' This reflects claims made by others, such as Ballweg (1992: 755), who claims that women will feel better if they educate themselves about their disease and take responsibility for managing the illness. Referring, for example, to women with endometriosis as 'consumers', Cox, Ski, Wood, et al. (2003a) argued that there exist 'a range of options available for the management of endometriosis, and consumers need to be made aware of all of these'. Other studies have also suggested the importance of women becoming educated about their bodies and the condition. In doing so, it is claimed, 'The more women understand, the more responsible they become for their actions and, as such, the physician does not have to "take all the blame"' (Cox, Ski, Wood, et al. 2003a: 207). This would be beneficial, it was suggested, for it would give consumers 'hope and a sense of control' (Cox, Ski, Wood, et al. 2003a: 208) over their situation. In much of this work, it is not always apparent what references to women 'taking charge' of their health means, nor precisely what becoming more 'assertive' or taking 'control' involves. Moreover, it is not always clear how or why getting off 'the medical roundabout' would be 'empowering', nor – perhaps more importantly – what the authors understand 'empowerment' to mean. In existing literature, certain actions on the part of women – such as reading about the disease – appear to be characterised as 'taking charge', after which 'taking charge' is assumed to be 'empowering', and 'empowerment' is positioned as almost self-evidently desirable. The assumption here seems to be that because many women will have had negative experiences with biomedicine, 'self-care' is both *inevitable* and *preferable.* The problem for many women with endometriosis, however, is not necessarily one of *excessive* medical care (implied by notion that it is beneficial to get off the 'medical roundabout') – it is, rather, a lack of *any* or *any meaningful* medical care. Women, we will recall, experience delays of 9 years, on average, to diagnosis (Phillips and Motta 2000: 6; Ballweg 2003a: 355) and many women want more, not less, medical intervention. This complexity is often overlooked in academic work on the disease. In their support for self-care, then, academics have tended to explicitly endorse a neoliberal philosophy of healthcare and the model of the responsible, rational, informed consumer-citizen that figures so prominently in self-help discourses.

As to *why* women became more 'proactive', only a few explanations have been offered in previous work.[2] On the one hand, women were said to be frustrated by the lack of information and support they received from health professionals (Cox, Henderson, Anderson, et al. 2003b: 7). In the main, however, it was suggested that women who 'managed to take control of their lives did so because of duress' (Cox, Henderson, Wood, et al. 2003c: 67). They had, that is, 'no choice in the end' (Cox, Henderson, Anderson, et al. 2003b: 7). Unfortunately, the two Cox et al. studies (2003b, 2003c) do not stipulate what duress means in this context, how women are the victims of duress, from whom or what this pressure emerges, nor why it is that women have no other choice but to become proactive patients. Curiously, then, previous research seems to be suggesting that women

---

2   This is not a problem confined to the aforementioned studies. Studies of people who suffer from other conditions report evidence of subjects becoming responsible or proactive in their care but have little to say about the processes involved. In a study of indigenous Australians affected with HIV, for example, Newman, Bonar, Greville, et al. (2007: 578) reported their research participants 'describing a kind of "responsibilisation" in the period after their HIV diagnosis' and suggested that 'HIV infection is conceived as a turning point in the "journey" of taking greater responsibility for your health'. Despite the fact that responsibilisation was a central issue in that study, the authors said nothing else about how or why responsibilisation might occur beyond the suggestion that being diagnosed with a condition provokes responsibilised behaviour.

become proactive (at least partly) through forced coercion of some kind, but that becoming more proactive is ultimately positive. Unfortunately, this literature also produces a confused version of women's agency, one in which women figure as both the victims of power and as empowered. Of course it is possible that women are both of these things (and that they are neither). The point is that however one interprets these findings, existing studies raise many more questions than they answer. Perhaps most of all, we need to develop a better appreciation of what greater responsibility actually entails, and how we might understand women's responsibilising turn. Recent literature on responsibility, freedom and power provides a broad platform from which to examine these questions.

Responsibility, Freedom and Medical Power

Medical power is a topic of considerable interest to sociologists and scholars of science and technology studies. Some of the best-known sociological work on medical power emerged in the 1970s. In the work of Zola (1972), for instance, it was claimed that medicine is one of society's foremost institutions of social control, and that medicine plays a central function in the classification and management of deviance. According to Zola's approach, medicine has a largely normalising effect, through first, the classification of certain bodies, bodily processes and behaviours as pathological, abnormal and undesirable, and second, through the promotion of medical methods to 'correct' those deviant bodies. The work of Zola and his contemporaries (e.g. Illich 1976; Friedson 1970) is therefore underpinned by a very particular understanding of power. Power is conceptualised as an object that is possessed by a minority (doctors) and imposed, from the 'top down' on the few (such as homosexuals, women, and the 'disabled'). One example of how this might be achieved is through the process of 'medicalisation', a practice whereby ordinary processes of the body (such as menstruation and pregnancy) come to be defined as 'medical problems' requiring medical management (Nettleton 1995: 27). There is an implicit assumption in much of this work that patients are passive and vulnerable in the face of authoritative medical practitioners. This understanding of the relationship between medical professionals and their patients is broadly referred to as an 'orthodox' approach (Lupton 1997).

The orthodox approach to medicine, while still valid in some respects, has been subject to sustained criticism in recent years and become less germane over time. The assumption, for example, that medical interactions are always already negative is now recognised as an overly simplistic approach. Many people, of course, do not experience medical encounters as problematic – indeed, for many, encounters with biomedicine are positive experiences. There are also problems with the assumption that doctors operate in a more or less uniform way, and that patients figure as universally vulnerable or lack agency (Bury 1997; Armstrong 1984). To the extent that women are one of the foremost 'victims' of medical power and medicalisation, the orthodox approach also constructs women as inherently vulnerable and powerless in medical settings. This is a version of agency that simply cannot be sustained. In addition, Mike Bury (1997: 100–107) has made the point that that the orthodox perspective on biomedicine is increasingly irrelevant in the West, as the position and prestige of doctors has been gradually eroded over time. The emergence of the Internet is often cited as evidence of this, insofar as it allows patients greater opportunities to engage with alternative medical information and to potentially challenge medical authority.

Michel Foucault's work is perhaps the best-known counterpoint to the orthodox approach. His work is underpinned by a radically different conceptualisation of power, one in which power is understood to function through an 'infinitesimal' number of 'mechanisms' (Foucault 1980b: 99). According to Foucault, power is neither localised nor possessed by a limited number of actors – such as doctors (Foucault 1980a: 59–60). Instead, famously, he declared that power could be found 'everywhere', as a force that operated through individuals. A particular title or set of qualifications was neither essential nor inherent to Foucault's concept of power; the point instead was that power flows through a range of individuals and institutions, including doctors, self-help groups, friends, family and, importantly, the patient themselves (Foucault 1980c: 142).

In his later works, Foucault (1988: 18) collapsed many of his original ideas together with his conception of 'technologies' that operate with regards the subject. In *Technologies of the Self*, published posthumously, he outlined four main types of technologies, including technologies of the self which:

> permit individuals to effect by their own means or with the help of others a certain number of operations on their own bodies and souls, thoughts, conduct, and way of being, so as to transform themselves in order to attain a certain state of happiness, purity, wisdom, perfection, or immortality. (Foucault 1988: 18)

According to this approach, one of the main ways in which power 'functions' is through practices of self-regulation (Foucault 1977). Self-regulation may take many forms – as the quote above implies. It may involve, for example, injunctions to patients to take a more active role in their own care, or to manage and monitor themselves in diverse ways. The Foucauldian scholar Graham Burchell (1996: 29) has described this productive approach to action as one that:

> Involves "offering" individuals and collectivities active involvement in action to resolve the kind of issues hitherto held to be the responsibility of authorized governmental agencies … This might be described as a new form of "responsibilization" corresponding to the new forms in which the governed are encouraged, freely and rationally, to conduct themselves.

This can be contrasted to a more repressive model of action, which sees individuals as the victims of duress or coercion. The Foucauldian approach to responsibilisation is thus concerned with the infinitesimal mechanisms by which power circulates, as well as the 'productive' dimensions of such power. It may involve, for instance, processes whereby individuals are enjoined to become 'self-actualizing' (Fullagar 2002: 72) and desiring subjects who actively take responsibility for their own health care.

In recent years, Nikolas Rose has written extensively on the relationship between action, responsibility, freedom and choice. His explication of this relationship offers important insights that might help us to understand processes of responsibilisation in the present case. Freedom, according to Rose, is often regarded as the antithesis of government, insofar as the term is used by most political theorists (Rose 1999). Traditionally freedom has been imagined as:

> the absence of coercion or domination; it was a condition in which the essential subjective will of an individual, a group or a people could express itself and was not silenced, subordinated or enslaved by an alien power. (Rose 1999: 1)

But Rose, borrowing from Foucault's work on governmentality, argues for a different understanding of freedom. He argues that freedom is not the antithesis of government, but one of the central pillars and main resources of government. Freedom, in the sense Rose conceives of it, is a fundamental form of government, embracing 'the ways in which one might be urged and educated to bridle one's own passions, to control one's own instincts, to govern oneself' (Rose 1999: 3). Rose argues that citizens are not simply permitted to 'be free' – they are expected to be. As 'personal life becomes a matter of freedom of choice' (Rose 1999: 65) the enterprising, self-regulating subject, whose private conduct is centred around 'techniques of self-understanding and self-mastery' (Rose 1999: 69) becomes increasingly obliged to manage and develop themselves, to make appropriate and rational choices. In a classic statement on the nature of freedom as obligation, Rose (1996: 17) writes:

> The forms of freedom we inhabit today are intrinsically bound to a regime of subjectification in which subjects are not merely "free to choose", but obliged to be free, to understand and enact their lives in terms of choice under conditions that systematically limit the capacities of many to shape their own destiny.

For present purposes, this is important in two ways. First, conduct is not seen to develop within a repressive context but instead, precisely because of the (apparent) absence of coercion. And secondly, within this context, the opportunities for surveillance of the individual actually increase. Rose's analysis of freedom views enterprising subjects as participating in an ethos of government that differs from a state-imposed or coercive form of governance but which is no less powerful in its effects on the subject. Here, this might mean that women with endometriosis are obliged to be 'free' – but free in the (somewhat ironic) sense of self-governing. Insofar as responsible and enterprising citizens have the 'freedom' to do so, they are obliged to utilise the opportunities generated by that freedom. In this sense, women become proactive not only because they have 'no choice' (Cox, Henderson, Anderson, et al. 2003b). They do so precisely because they have choices. Taking control of one's own situation is an exercise of agency, but most likely an exercise of agency in *a particular way and in accordance with a particular rationality.* Burchell (1996: 24) would call this 'the proper use of liberty'.

Women, Gender and Citizenship

Although I consider Nikolas Rose's work around responsibility, freedom and choice to be very useful, there are at least two important limitations that I want to briefly touch upon. First, and most importantly, Rose's work largely ignores gender, in the sense that the obligation to be free is portrayed as something that applies more or less universally to citizens.[3] This invites some difficulties because, for instance, men and women are subject to different kinds of obligations and injunctions, and to differing degrees. The imperative to care, for instance, is constituted as one of the main obligations of femininity, and differs markedly from the ways men are often asked, invited or expected to 'care' (Stacey 1997). Feminist political theorists might also challenge the suggestion that women's experiences of 'citizenship' are similar to men's (Jones 1998: 221) or the idea that women figure as citizens at all. Many feminists have highlighted problematic aspects of the relationship between the body and citizenship (see Bacchi and Beasley 2002) and it has been argued that 'citizens act as embodied subjects whose interests reflect their biological and psychosocial reality' (Jones 1998: 230).[4] What this all means is that women with endometriosis may be obliged to govern themselves, but that these obligations may emerge at least partly in gendered ways. They may be obliged to act, for instance, because they are women, women whose 'freedom' is constituted through the expectations attached to them as menstruating, reproductive bodies. The activities women undertake also undoubtedly serve to perform gender (as well, perhaps, as race, culture, disability, and the like). Without considering gender, then, Rose's work ends up neglecting the various ways that obligations and practices pertaining to women may be gendered, as well as the way that such practices 'kick back',

---

3   Although in more recent years he has considered gender more explicitly (e.g. Rose 2007).

4   Jones (1998: 221) summarises feminist critiques of citizenship as follows: 'Not only do women lack the full complement of citizenship "rights" included in citizenship, but also the conceptualization of citizenship in these systems – the characteristics, qualities, attributes, behavior, and identity of those who are regarded as full members of the political community – is derived from a set of values, experiences, modes of discourse, rituals, and practices that both explicitly privileges men and the "masculine" and excludes women and the "female".'

by which I mean produce and reproduce women, gender, femininity, feminine forms of obligation, and so on.

In what follows, I explore the way that self-care, responsibility and gender play out for women with endometriosis. As will quickly become apparent, women regularly embark upon journeys of self-discovery and self-management after diagnosis, and they often engage in activities that might be broadly understood as forms of self-care. It is too simple, however, to characterise this as emerging through 'duress', or as self-evidently 'empowering' and positive. It is also too simple to characterise these practices as forms of the largely universal obligations or duties of free 'citizenship', following Rose. Instead, women's practices reflect and reproduce gender in ways that are both familiar and concerning. I argue that women's practices tend to be dominated by three main themes:

1. A sense of themselves as inherently irrational and dysfunctional when menstruating – a notion that I refer to as the 'monstrous feminine'. The monster is a figure consistent with historic understandings of women as anomalous (as compared to men), irrational and excessively emotional. Women perform themselves as the monstrous feminine while menstruating but this figure may appear right across the month for those women who report extended menstrual symptoms, and where such symptoms are attributed to the disease;
2. Women perform an ontological separation of self and subject that is similar to the kind that I described in Chapter 3, but with variations and contradictions that are both subtle and significant. Insofar as women perform this separation, control of the unruly 'body' or 'self' emerges as both a possibility and an obligation. This is a gendered phenomenon linked to the sense of one's underlying monstrousness;
3. A model of one's own subjectivity as disordered and multiple, with women's lives characterised by a desire to live more authentically and rationally. Women's 'responsibilising' turn emerges partly in response to this disordered and inappropriate subjectivity and is at least partially an attempt to position oneself as authentic, rational and ordered.

In what follows, I want to focus, first, on the process of being enjoined towards self-care. After this I examine how self-analysis and self-care practices surface in women's accounts of living with the disease and what they might mean. I then consider how these instances surface particular notions of responsibility, subjectivity and ontology and what these mean for the women concerned.

Becoming a 'Responsible' Subject

As with earlier studies, most of the women I interviewed reported a greater 'responsibilising' turn following their endometriosis diagnosis. This occurs for a range of reasons; many women, for instance, felt frustrated with mainstream medicine, especially those who had negative experiences or lengthy delays to diagnosis. Some women felt the need to try and take more 'control' of their bodies because they deemed there to be little alternative. In a number of instances, doctors were blunt in their assessments about their future prospects, telling women that because little was known about the disease, very little could be done. Importantly, women became more pro-active in relation to their health for other reasons too, including a concern about their behaviour in the face of the disease and/or the impact that their behaviour was having on other people. These issues have not been examined in the previous literature. According to Sarah, aged 44, the most important thing in the post-diagnostic period was going to be her 'attitude'. After talking with her doctors, she reached the conclusion that the main symptom of her endometriosis – menstrual pain – was primarily:

> *mental* because the gynaecologist I ended up sticking with for most of my operations, he said to me initially when I said "I want a hysterectomy, I want it gone, I can't handle this anymore", he said to me he could put me on a pill – this is interesting and he is probably right – he could put me on a pill that I think is going to help me or put me on a sugar pill and he would guarantee I would come back and I would say I would feel so much better. Because he said "A lot of it is psychological". And I said "You are damn right, you are damn right" … He is right, a lot of it is.

Through the clinical interaction, Sarah is invited to think of her pain as largely 'mental' and to see herself as having the capacity to act upon or even control her symptoms. Juxtaposed against the 'official' biomedical line – that endometriosis is a disease of uncertain ætiology with no known cure – Sarah's physician produces her as a potentially agentive subject. To the extent that Sarah's understanding of menstrual pain reflects that of her treating doctor (as probably 'psychological'), she is both producing and reproducing menstrual pain as a primarily psychogenic or psychosomatic phenomenon. Through this encounter, Sarah enacts herself as not just *an* agent, but as the *main* agent in relation to the disease; she seems to understand her doctor to be saying that gynaecological medicine has little role to play here (although whether he is arguing for a greater degree of medicalisation via psychological medicine is unclear). Nevertheless, as later aspects of my interview with Sarah revealed, the central figure in the post-diagnostic phase is not going to be her doctor: it is, quite clearly, her.

Sarah, like many other women, experienced severe pain and mood swings; she understood these mood swings as both a 'symptom' of the disease and an 'effect' of the hormonal medication she was taking to treat the endometriosis. As she explained:

> I had a feeling, and I ended up saying to this third doctor I went to, to say "please help me, something is wrong with me. I'm not normally this crazy. I cry,

[I'm] topsy-turvy". I said, "I feel like walking out and just jumping in front of a bus and saying, 'Thanks very much, been a great life, see you later'" ... And my husband kept saying "what the bloody hell is the matter with you? You are driving us all insane". And I was. And I said, "I don't know. I don't know why I am doing this. I have no idea" ... So he had had enough as well. He had to go through I guess every month I would just sit there and be a basket case: "Don't talk to me. Don't speak to me.". I'd settle myself on the couch, I'd just get up – heat up my beanbags in the microwave, come back down, sit back down again.

In this account, Sarah's burgeoning ethic of self-care is constituted partially through a sense of obligation to others, triggered by the belief that she was 'crazy' and a 'basket case'. The relational aspect of self-care was also a key trigger for another woman in the study, Maddy, who explained that the 'biggest motivator' to start managing the condition herself was:

actually [my] problems with relationships. I rarely spoke to any of my friends, when I spoke to my parents or sister all I did was whinge and my sex life with my husband was non-existent. I didn't like the person I was becoming and I felt that a lot of it had to do with how I was dealing with my illness. Therefore I had to make some serious changes. My main concerns were in regards to my husband, I didn't have any energy or time to give to us. All I ever did was whinge at him, either because I was in pain and unhappy or because I was moody and emotional and therefore everything he did was the wrong thing. We hardly ever had sex, either I was too tired or in too much pain or just didn't feel like it, we never went out, we never saw our friends, I basically had no interest in us, I was just too focused on me and my problems.

Writing about the experiences of cancer patients, Jackie Stacey (1997: 197) argued that women are often subject to 'an imperative to care', an imperative bound up with notions of femininity:

This sense of obligation can be seen as an extension of the already well-established duties of femininity: the duty to care for the self, building on the feminine conscience to care for others (as wives, mothers, teachers, nurses, and so on). Building on the construction of femininity as responsible for the family, for the nation and for civilisation itself, the cancer patient is addressed through the further burden of being directly (and sometimes solely) responsible for their own health and illness.

Many of the women I interviewed emphasised these relational elements in the emergence of a more proactive and 'responsibilised' approach towards the disease. This obligation is often enacted via women's descriptions of themselves as inherently irrational and dysfunctional when menstruating. To the extent that emotions are one of the main parts of the 'problem' requiring management, then, the control of emotions became a central cause for concern among women, and a central target in self-care practices.

Managing the 'Monstrous' Self

Many women with endometriosis viewed themselves as 'monstrous', seeing their behaviour as largely problematic, especially during menstruation. This comprises several elements: first, women understood themselves as emotionally dysfunctional and irrational. Even when their 'errant' emotionality was understood as a symptom of their disease, or of their treatment, women positioned this as something that needed to be controlled, and as something for which *they* were ultimately responsible. As Maddy explained, for instance, the belief that her disease made her a 'monster' was a major factor in her investigating options in relation to diet and lifestyle:

> I am just an evil monster a few days a month. And so [I thought] if I could do *something* to control that, then great. I think about ripping it all out sometimes, just getting it all out of there [and having a hysterectomy]. My family have often wanted me to rip it all out, just to get it over and done with.

In this account, Maddy constitutes herself as an 'evil monster', expressing a need to rationalise and control that aspect of her 'self' that she considers monstrous. Despite her realisation that 'being moody is part and parcel of the condition and I shouldn't beat myself up over it', Maddy was adamant that she would not use this as a justification for poor behaviour:

> You have got to try and learn to deal with it and you have got to, I mean, you can't use the endometriosis as an excuse to fly off the handle.

Here, Maddy seeks to repudiate problematic emotional behaviours typically associated with women, including moodiness, excessive emotionality, irrationality and weakness. The fact that women who have been diagnosed with a disease may try to construct themselves as strong, rational, responsible and pro-active is neither novel nor, perhaps, unsurprising. In work examining the experiences of people living with HIV, for instance, Deborah Lupton (1993) argues that when citizens undertake to care for themselves, their actions should not merely be understood as instances of self-management but as attempts to simultaneously demonstrate that they have adopted a responsible approach to their health problems. Among women with endometriosis, there is a distinctly gendered element to this behaviour, however, insofar as women attribute elements of their personality and behaviour to the disease, and insofar as these patterns are further understood as connected to menstruation. In these ways, then, the post-diagnostic period becomes a time in which women reflect upon and produce themselves as irrational subjects with problematic behavioural traits that emerge *because of* endometriosis. This is perhaps best demonstrated through Barbara, another woman who understood her 'self' as problematic, and who engaged with a range of practices after diagnosis. One of the things she had done was develop an approach, together with her gynaecologist where she would menstruate just twice a year. This was designed not to alleviate her experience of pain, but to avoid:

> The alternative, to have my period every month, and just trying to explain to everybody why you turn into Satan for three or four days.

Here, Barbara performs her subjectivity as 'fractured': split between a more calm, stable and rational self and an alternative, irrational and disordered one that materialises when she menstruates. On these days, she literally becomes someone (or something) else. The solution, as she explained:

> ... the way I've essentially developed it, is, I'm only allowed two periods a year. Um, I have to continue to take my pill straight through, and when I do get my periods I tend to get cluster migraines as well 'cos I haven't had it for a while.

To the extent that endometriosis is symbolically adjacent to 'excessive' menstruation and femininity, as discussed in earlier chapters, the post-diagnostic period becomes an opportunity for women like Barbara to correct the very essence of the problem: menstruation and femininity 'itself'. The need to repudiate the symbolically 'feminine' appeared to be a central concern to women, especially after diagnosis, and is a major precipitating factor in their practices of self-care. Both Barbara and Maddy's accounts reflect and reproduce cultural constructions of women as inherently 'monstrous'. As Jane Ussher argues in *Managing the Monstrous Feminine*, women have long been constituted as monsters.[5] This process extends at least as far back as Aristotle, who believed that:

> Woman is literally a monster: a failed and botched male who is only born female due to an excess of moisture and of coldness during the process of conception. (Ussher 2006: 1)

Rosi Braidotti (1994: 81) argues that the positioning of women as monstrous stems from the constructed difference between women and men:

> Woman, as sign of difference, is monstrous. If we define the monster as a bodily entity that is anomalous and deviant vis-à-vis the norm, then we can argue that the female body shares with the monster the privilege of bringing out a unique blend of fascination and horror.

---

5   These ideas have also been explored by Julia Kristeva (1982) and Barbara Creed (2007) among others. See also Ussher (2003).

It is this sense of woman – as both fascinating and horrifying – that Ussher suggests has legitimated the medical management of women. But what we see here is women constituting themselves as literally monstrous: as anomalous, deviant and horrible. These findings bear similarities to those in a study conducted by Karin Martin (2003), who interviewed 26 women about their experiences of giving birth in order to determine 'the internalised technologies or sense of gender that women bring with them to birth' (Martin 2003: 56). She found that women regulated their own behaviour during labour in a way that complied with and reproduced social 'norms' (Martin 2003: 54). Women were 'compelled from within to act in gender-normative ways' by expending a great degree of:

> Energy on taking care of others and obeying gendered social norms about politeness while they were in the middle of a profound physical experience that takes considerable energy, agency and willpower. (2003: 69)

Martin's study demonstrates one way in which women regulate their behaviour through a process of internalising technologies of gender, by which I mean 'knowledge, discourses, and practices' about the way they understand that women should ideally behave (2003: 56). Women with endometriosis also sought to control their emotional responses to chronic illness and to the debilitating experience of menstrual difficulties in ways that they deemed gender appropriate.

Sarah, whose story I introduced earlier, struggled with severe menstrual pain. In our interview, she reflected upon her experiences of menstrual pain as a school student, a pain that would often result in her spending the entire day in the sick bay:

> [When I was younger] because my mum couldn't understand it, my sister had none of it and here I am looking like the one who is sooking all the time and taking time off school. I used to spend so much time in sick bay it was embarrassing and it was like once a month in sick bay and it was like "She must have her period again" ... I used to go in and this is Marie, the one who looked after the girls' problems. That's what we called it back then. She used to bring me a bucket, because I used to feel really nauseous and would be just curled up in a ball and just thought "Oh". Because we lived in – to get to school we had to catch a bus and a bus home – so once you got to school you couldn't get home. My mother didn't drive, dad worked, so I had to spend the day in horrible sickbay on a stretcher bed until I got back home and just crawled into bed and just stayed there.

In our interview, Sarah's approach of just crawling 'into bed and just staying there' could be contrasted with how she now approached her menstrual cycle:

> I don't like to sound, like a lot of women are sooks, they are hypochondriacs, they can't help themselves. Guys are when they are sick, but women can sort of, I don't know, we sometimes seem to bitch and whinge about *everything* ...

> My motto [now] is if you are sick, get up and have a shower, you'll feel a lot
> better, moving right along, just get on with it.

In this account, Sarah seeks to draw a distinction between her past and present
behaviour in two ways. First, following Fraser (2004), she performs herself as
a responsible subject by contrasting her presently positive and more measured
approach to menstrual pain ('moving right along, just get on with it') with the
negative and inactive approach she enacted as a younger woman ('[I] just crawled
into bed and just stayed there'). The emphasis in these excerpts is upon Sarah's
transformation into a newly responsible subject, one that has abandoned her
previously lazy practices. Secondly, Sarah contrasts her own emotionally restrained
approach in recent times to the apparently problematic reactions of 'sooks' and
'hypochondriacs'. Through her repudiation of both her own previous conduct and
the irrational conduct of others, Sarah seeks to position herself as a responsible
subject outside the 'domain of the abject' (Butler 1993: 3), a space occupied by
men and women who 'whinge', 'bitch' and 'sook' about illness. Although she
positions men as capable of problematic emoting, she understands this to happen
in very limited circumstances (when they are 'sick'), whereas women have the
ability to 'bitch and whinge about everything'. It is unclear whether Sarah actually
recognises herself, like the men she mentions, as 'sick', nor whether she permits
herself to feel or express emotions as a result. Drawing a distinction along sharply
gendered lines, Sarah instead constitutes herself as naturally prone to excessive
and irrational emotionality. Importantly, she also celebrates the way she has
become a newly rational and responsible subject through learning to contain these
aspects of her 'nature'. These themes – the constitution of oneself as a responsible,
emotionally restrained and rational subject – appeared repeatedly throughout my
discussions with women when talking about the post-diagnostic phase of their
illness. In the next section I look more closely at the accounts of three women
for whom self-care was an important practice, exploring what taking greater
responsibility for oneself actually involves, and how such practices function,
especially in respect to gender.

Authenticity, Ontology and the Psychology of Self-care

Alice

Alice was 35 years old and lived with her partner, David. She first experienced the
symptoms of the condition aged 30 and was diagnosed in the same year. In the two
years following diagnosis, Alice had laparoscopic surgery on five occasions and had
been unable to engage in any paid work because of the severity of her symptoms.
In this period her health rapidly declined and she became very fatigued, with a
subsequent diagnosis of chronic fatigue syndrome. Alice had become very active
in exploring other treatment options, reading self-help books, and had attended a

self-help group (although she did not feel she obtained much insight there). She engaged with Chinese medicine, adopted a macrobiotic diet and tried acupuncture. Like most other women in the study, then, Alice's post-diagnostic experiences were characterised by experimentation with a diverse range of treatments. Her practice required considerable self-discipline, as she 'allowed' herself only small amounts of certain foods, eliminating others entirely and regularly taking 'revolting' herbs and food that she thought was 'disgusting', including a drink that was made from squirrel faeces. Her healthcare routine was also incredibly time-consuming: 'my whole day was boiling herbs, having a shower and going back to bed' (Alice).

Alongside all of this, Alice became more interested in processes of self-reflection, yoga, meditation and contemplation after her formal diagnosis. Rather than trying to control her body, or fix the disease, Alice's emphasis was upon *relinquishing* any desire to control the self or body. She described this as a liberating experience:

> It's more for me about letting go of control … My feeling about the whole [disease] in general is that there are lots of different theories and lots of different treatments, but I think whether you get to the bottom of it or not doesn't matter. But I think there is always a deeper reason for illness, an emotional, or spiritual reason, or something. And if you look at it that way you don't necessarily have to fix it or even find out how to fix it. It has helped me, in terms of being able to accept that there is a reason [for disease].

In this account, Alice suggests that there is likely to be a 'deeper' explanation for her having developed endometriosis, thus invoking psychological disease explanations that I have touched upon in earlier chapters. Once the underlying psychological basis for the disease is discovered, it did not necessarily have to be fixed, dealt with, controlled, or overcome. In this sense, Alice's approach to self-care seems to differ from that of the women described in the Cox et al. (2003a, 2003b, 2003c) studies examined earlier. She doesn't consider herself to be 'taking charge' of her body or in 'control' of the disease. Indeed, she is actively concerned to *avoid* taking control, to the extent that she might be expected to do so. In spite of Alice's apparent disinterest in trying to either 'fix' or 'control' her disease, just days after our interview she headed to the South American jungle to spend six months in the forest. The aim of her trip, she later explained, was to explore the 'deeper reasons' for her illness:

> I don't really want to dwell on what I see as being, I guess, the negative side of [endometriosis]. I know for me I feel there is a deeper reason for illness I'd rather look into than why my physical – I'm interested in focusing on the deeper stuff.

The focus of the South American trip, like much of the work she had been undertaking after diagnosis, was in trying to uncover what she referred to as her 'real essence'. As part of this process, Alice was committed to 'stripping away' her ego and 'letting go' of everything that she had held on to, everything that she had thought of as her '*self*'.

Although Alice does not understand a desire for control as a motivating factor in her self-care practices, she is, nevertheless, searching for something. She wanted to:

> let go of all the crap or a lot of the crap – not all of the crap – but you know, like, in the way I want to talk to people, it's like the real essence comes out.

The notion of 'authenticity' is central to Alice's self-care practice. Here, for example, she performs subjectivity as multiple, divided between an authentic and inauthentic self, through references to the 'real essence' that lay underneath 'all the crap'. As I understand this, Alice is articulating a desire to achieve, through various practices, a more 'authentic' version of subjectivity – one that she understands as being connected in some way to the development of the disease. It is unclear whether Alice feels she has 'lost' touch with this authentic self, or whether she has never actualised an 'authentic' form of subjecthood.[6] The search for the authentic self is common among individuals who have been diagnosed with a chronic illness. Jackie Stacey, for instance, has identified authenticity as an important theme in cancer discourses, whereby:

> This retrieval of lost or hidden knowledge about the self is seen as central to the healing process. It is not about becoming someone else, but rather *becoming who you are*. The real you, who knows of a more caring and nurturing existence from the past, needs to return, take control and show the misguided parts of you the way forward. (1997: 197; emphasis in original)

---

6   The notion of the 'lost' self is well known in sociological literature on chronic illness but here I am using it in a different sense to the way it is usually deployed within sociology. For example, Kathy Charmaz (1983) conceptualises chronic illness as producing a fundamental 'loss of self'. This is problematic, I suggest, because it implies a singular, prior and stable 'self' that is disrupted with the advent of chronic illness. This is problematic for at least three reasons. First – and at the risk of labouring the point – subjectivity does not exist prior to its materialisation or performance through various acts, practices etc. Secondly, the notion of a 'lost self' suggests that subjectivity is both singular and interior to the subject rather than pluralistic and diverse (or perhaps more accurately, multiple). Thirdly, although Charmaz appears to recognise the *productive* function of illness – in a sense that might be considered broadly Foucauldian – her work also implies that chronic illness acts upon the fixed/prior subject in ways that are largely negative, unsettling and disruptive. This is apparent in her depiction of a 'loss' of self, a phrase that broadly signals illness as a deficit. These descriptions deny the positive dimensions of illness for some people and the performative dimensions of subjecthood. Finally, it implies that individuals respond (more or less) uniformly to the challenges thrown up by chronic illness, without acknowledging the variations that may be produced through different types of chronic illness.

Stacey argues that the self is positioned as having multiple components, where one more authentic 'part' is constructed as being responsible for looking after the 'rest'. Alice's 'New Age' ethic reflects and reproduces a very similar version of subjectivity – one in which the subject's obligation is to develop a more 'authentic' relationship with oneself.[7]

Some theorists (e.g. Lupton 2003) have argued that the New Age philosophy of health and illness involves a rejection of the traditional Cartesian mind/body dualism, whereby the body and self are positioned as ontologically distinct. On the contrary, however, I read Alice's practice as both 'New Age' and closely aligned to Cartesian dualism, insofar as she emphasises the capacity of her (ontologically separate and superior) self to know the body (because the body's disease is a symptom of the inauthentic 'self'). Alice understands herself as being capable of controlling her body, it is just that she is not necessarily willing to do so. In this sense, Alice's account of living with endometriosis reproduces the ontological separation of self/body that circulates in self-help literature, but she engages with the obligations that attach to this version of ontology in quite a novel way. This does not mean, however, that Alice isn't concerned with identifying and correcting any problems of the self or body. As her account makes clear, she is driven by a desire to uncover her 'authentic' self. In so doing, Alice enacts a dualism of authentic/inauthentic subjectivity that both reflects and reproduces traditional forms of dichotomous thinking. As I noted earlier in this book, for instance, women and femininity have historically figured as inauthentic and irrational, whereas men and masculinity figure as authentic and rational. To the extent that Alice's self-care practices involve an attempt to live her life more 'authentically' and 'rationally', then, she is seeking access to a version of subjecthood that is both valorised and traditionally reserved for men. Her self-care practices are therefore a partially gendered phenomenon: a reflection of traditional understandings of gender, and a reproduction of them.

Yolanda

In many ways Alice's philosophy of disease shared similarities with Yolanda. Yolanda was a 41-year-old psychotherapist who lived with her husband Sebastian. She was diagnosed with endometriosis not long before her 22nd birthday, around eight years after the onset of symptoms. After initial diagnostic surgery, Yolanda's doctors placed her on hormonal drug treatments, but she experienced very severe side effects, including depression and mood swings. She explored complementary and alternative therapies, including psychotherapy, and found them to be more

---

7   This is a characteristic typical of those associated with the New Age movement more generally (Possamai 2000). In Adam Possamai's qualitative exploratory study of New Agers, he discovered that '83 per cent of my informants locate the inner self as the arbiter of the spiritual quest' and that New Agers demonstrate a form of subjectivism in which 'one should find one's own path' (2000: 369).

beneficial than mainstream medical options. At the time of our interview she was virtually pain free and pregnant with her first child. After being diagnosed with endometriosis, Yolanda became determined to manage the disease herself. Shortly after her diagnosis she resolved to:

> do something. There was nothing [the doctors] could really do for me, so [I thought] I have got to find out for myself.

Around this time Yolanda was introduced to the concept of spiritual healing. She described spiritual healing as opening 'up a whole new world to me that I had never really discovered before and knew was out there'. She began to study dreams and to explore her mind. It was during this period that Yolanda was exposed to mystical teachings about menstruation. She read about the way the menstrual cycle was understood in other cultures and through contemplation and meditation, she eventually uncovered a causal explanation for endometriosis that made sense to her:

> Because I always had so much pain with menstruation, I really felt "Oh God what is this, is this some kind of curse?" So there was that whole kind of thing – I don't know if you remember it – the curse of women? And I used to think to myself, you know it doesn't make any sense at all. So I would try and work that out in my mind and I couldn't come to terms with that theory at all. And so I started studying then some of the, I guess, the old Celtic Goddess mythology and European mythology, studied the native American tradition, which was very helpful, how they worked, the indigenous cultures, the rites of passage that are there for women when they first menstruate, that we obviously didn't experience in the West. But when they go through menopause and all the really important phases in a woman's life, it's interesting how the view of menstruation is very, very different to how we see it. So I really started working with my psyche and what was in my psyche and obviously my mother's own experience with menstruation hasn't been good, nor her mother's, so it's kind of come down again through the family system, which wasn't very healthy. So I really, really worked hard to shift my emphasis, start listening to my body, working with my cycle, taking a break … When I was ovulating, [I started] really tuning into my body and welcoming my period and that part of being a woman. And that was a huge shift for me.

For Yolanda, it was a matter of reconnecting the self and body and of seeking harmony with her menstrual cycle:

> it was almost like [the menstrual cycle] was something that was happening to me but wasn't a part of me. And because there was so much pain involved. I dreaded coming, dreaded [my period] and with all the pain I'd been through, just wanting it to be over, and so it was just something that was happening in my life, that I

really was like I was disassociated from it. And so what I tried to do was bring myself back into what was happening and working with the energy instead of fighting against it, pushing against it and that made a big difference. And I think hearing some of the myths in Ireland in particular and there are some beautiful stories around menstruation as well and which were in American Indian cultures as well and how it is honoured and how it is really about bringing that, that [menstruation] can be a blessing and not a curse. Just understanding that. That was big. I think then, that was what shifted whatever happened on a cellular level, the pain stopped. It took time though.

Here, Yolanda is practicing an ethic of self-care that performs the self and body as harmonious and fundamentally connected. This occurs through Yolanda's account of the menstrual cycle as a fundamental part of her 'self', as normal, natural and fundamentally her. In this sense I understand her approach as slightly different to Alice's, where a Cartesian separation between self and body is more clearly performed. When Yolanda speaks of her philosophy as one of 'working *with* my body', I understand her to be rejecting Cartesian dualism. This approach was taken into her work as a psychotherapist, where she dealt with women with a range of gynaecological problems, including endometriosis. Yolanda conducted classes for groups of women and encouraged them to explore their relationships with their menstrual cycles. In this work, she regularly enjoined her clients to seek a deeper understanding of the mind/spirit connection with the body and illness:

> that is one of the things I do – work with women who – that is what I do with women's groups here. We work around rites of passage for women and working with experience. We're working with women having difficulties with their cycle and so really exploring and talking about how they actually really feel about their womb, how they really feel about their cycle, what's going on with their period. It's just very interesting to be in a group with them and have them share because as women we don't normally talk about menstruation, it's still so taboo and I guess, that was part of the healing for me, was to take, start examining why it is taboo, why is it so secret, even amongst women, that we didn't talk about this part of our lives. And so expressing it, it's like it's not happening and that's exactly like it is on television, superwoman, she can climb a mountain when she has her periods. There is no sense of, actually your body is regenerating, you need to slow down, you need to look after yourself, other people look after you, which happens in other cultures, but not in the West. And that's not a sign of weakness, but a sign of strength, to give yourself that. So that's a really big shift in understanding all of the cycle as a woman. So that appeals to me, working on that shift in my psyche.

Like Alice, Yolanda's ethic is informed by both psychological and New Age philosophies of health and illness, especially those that emphasise illness as rooted in a woman's problematic relationship with 'femininity'. In Chapter 3 I considered some of the self-help literature around these issues, such as the work of Christiane Northrup (1998: 165) who emphasises an individualised approach to menstrual problems and the importance of women deciphering 'what her symptoms are trying to tell her'. Yolanda's practice reflects a similarly holistic mind/body/spirit approach to endometriosis, through a consideration of 'whatever might be going on for you ... opening up your mind to all of that'. Part of her practice is to counsel women and in the process of counselling them, she sought:

> I guess, to get a picture of what is going on in somebody's life as well, contributing factors to the illness as well and to getting worse or getting better too, what they can do for themselves.

Much like Alice, Yolanda is seeking an internal explanation for her menstrual problems, whilst encouraging the women she works with to develop their own methods – described as 'what they can do for themselves' – to resolve the problem, once the underlying cause of the problem had been identified. In Yolanda's classes the self is encouraged to interrogate its relation to the body (as well as to itself). In this way, Yolanda oscillates between a reiteration of the Cartesian dualism and a rejection of it.

Of particular interest is the fact that, like Alice, Yolanda understands self-transformation as a desirable and achievable goal. On more than one occasion, she explained that her health management practice involved, primarily, 'working with my attitude, changing my attitude'. For example, when Yolanda experienced discomfort or pain upon menstruation, she saw it as her body's way of telling her 'self' that she was working too hard:

> I think this is something that a lot of us choose, especially working hard with your career. We keep going, period or not and you keep pushing and you don't actually listen to your body and take time out when you need to.

This vigilant attention to the body and to her attitude towards her menstrual cycle continued even after Yolanda believed her endometriosis symptoms had alleviated:

> I really work with that still, I work with my psychotherapy, it is still very important. As I said, my [life] coach and I have continued with that, so that hasn't stopped at all.

Like the other women whose stories I have examined in this chapter, then, Yolanda's post-diagnostic practices are characterised by a pursuit of an authentic, rational and ordered self. Although I have suggested that Yolanda's understanding of the self/body relation is primarily one of interconnectedness and harmony, the self is ultimately positioned as superior to – and capable of mastering – the diseased body. In this respect, an ontological separation between self and body was a central motivating factor in Yolanda's self-care practice, as was a belief that disease was 'not normal' and that the self must be prepared to 'listen to the body' and change. The body and self are connected, that is, but only to the extent that a dysfunctional balance/relation between the two creates disease. Unlike Alice, then, Yolanda has a much stronger commitment to the notion that the self has the capacity to act upon the diseased body. Her self-care practices are firmly grounded in the understanding that she is responsible for her illness, and, in turn, for resolving it.

Chelsea

Chelsea was a 24-year-old research assistant with a science background who began experiencing symptoms of endometriosis around age 13. Chelsea's experiences of the disease were different to some of the other women I interviewed; having experienced severe pain and bowel problems from an early age, she had spent her teenage years bedbound, attending school when she could, and visiting a range of doctors. This period was dominated by an epistemological struggle to have her pain taken 'seriously' and resist the conclusion that the problem was 'all in her mind'. After being prescribed painkillers for several years, Chelsea was diagnosed with the disease via laparoscopy at the age of 18. After this initial operation, she underwent complicated follow-up surgery to remove endometriosis that had grown extensively into her bowels. For the last three years she had been on drug therapy and in a state of chemically induced 'menopause'. She still experienced a range of symptoms but the extent of her pain had dramatically declined. Even after diagnosis, Chelsea faced pressure from her treating doctors and members of her family to seek psychological help. Her main treating doctor once told her that her response to drug therapy was promising because he had not been sure, even after diagnosis, if the problem was mainly 'psychological'. Even though this event left her feeling 'really pissed off', Chelsea decided to follow medical advice to engage with psychiatric medicine thereafter, though she was reluctant to do so:

> I have had GPs who have insisted I go to see a psychiatrist ... constantly people trying to push me down the path of psychiatric answers ... I refused to see one for a long time and finally I did it just to shut everyone up.

> *Interviewer:* Was it a conscious decision on your part to go and see a psychiatrist to placate people?

> *Chelsea:* Pretty much just to placate people but I did it really quite, I was really pissed off. And [the psychiatrist] wrote in her report that [the problem] was everything that I had said to them anyway, so it worked out fine anyway, but I was really pissed off. She pissed me off. She wanted to know, I wanted to talk to her about this, the experiences of my illness and the symptoms I was having, and she wanted to talk to me about my family life, a very classic psychiatry thing which really drove me nuts. And in the end, I think she was just doing her job

and they have to take into account the whole spectrum and I appreciate that but it really annoyed me that I ended up at her because I had these peculiar symptoms and we weren't talking about them. We were talking about how I feel about my mum and dad. I actually feel very good about my mum and dad. I really don't want to pay $160 an hour to talk about my mum and dad.

When she finally attended a psychiatrist, she was keen to impress upon them that:

I fought really hard to have this taken seriously as a problem with my body rather than people just saying it is all in [my] head or something is wrong with you, and I feel that by being here, and on my records will be that I have seen a psychiatrist and I will just completely lose that battle. Because I think for women there is always that issue in medicine that if we can't come up with an explanation of what is going on, it is all in your imagination and you are screwy. And I felt like that was just going to haunt me when I had only just started to get away from that.

Referring again to the doctor who had doubted the extent to which the problem was physical, Chelsea explained that:

Ever since then I have been very conscious because [of] the psychological dimension ... of presenting myself always as "I have a *physical* problem that you need to help me with". Because of that first experience of him actually saying "I thought you were crazy, turned out you weren't".

How might we characterise Chelsea's approach to psychiatric treatment? Is it appropriate to describe her engagement with therapy as a form of self-care? Psychological therapy is often understood as such, but it is not clear that Chelsea is engaging with her psychiatrist in this way or for this reason. She seems, at the very least, ambivalent about psychiatry's treatment of women and worries that her treating psychiatrist will, like so many others, produce her as emotionally disordered and dysfunctional. How, then, might we understand Chelsea's agency in this encounter?

On the one hand, Chelsea enacts herself as a choosing subject, by explaining that the decision to finally engage with psychiatry was her choice alone. It is clear, however, that one of the reasons she understands herself to be engaging with therapy is to allay the concerns of others. Within the context of the clinical encounter, Chelsea seems less committed to obtaining emotional guidance or to exploring her relationship with menstruation (as Yolanda might), than she is in utilising that clinical space to establish her credentials as a stable and rational subject. Although it is possible to interpret what Chelsea is doing as agentive and a form of responsibilised self-care, the rationale for her engagement with psychiatric medicine is complicated. She is determined, that is, to establish epistemological and ontological credibility in the face of doubt that her problem was ever genuine –

or, perhaps more precisely, genuinely *physical*. In this sense, Chelsea's action needs to be understood as performing a more nuanced and complex version of agency than the kind articulated by either the Cox studies (2003a, 2003b, 2003c) or Rose (1999). Chelsea acts as a free subject, to be sure, but her agency is shaped in part by a desperate need to resist traditional gendered understandings of her body/self. Chelsea seems unable to draw any firm conclusions about what her engagement with psychiatric medicine ultimately achieves, however, thus flagging the sometimes unsatisfactory dimensions of the way self-care activities actually proceed. I will return to a consideration of these complexities at the conclusion of this chapter.

Chelsea engaged in a range of other activities after diagnosis, including dietary and other lifestyle changes. She described her behaviour as 'fastidious', and noted that people around her sometimes worried that her practices were 'over the top'. Because of this, as she explained at one point: 'My family think I am insane.' Her understanding of why she had come to manage her diet and lifestyle differed from the approach of Alice and Yolanda. It also differed from the findings in previous studies regarding how and why women become more pro-active in relation to their own disease (Ballweg 2003f; Cox, Ski, Wood, et al. 2003a; Cox, Henderson, Anderson, et al. 2003b; Cox, Henderson, Wood, et al. 2003c). As Chelsea explained:

> I never felt there was anything that I could really do at all that would control the growing of it or those kind of core things. I never looked at that as my responsibility to control it. It is just going to do what it is going to do. But it is more the kind of secondary symptoms, the digestion stuff that I have worked hard to control and that has been good, that has actually worked.

Although many aspects of Chelsea's engagement with mainstream medicine were negative, she was not necessarily hostile towards biomedicine as a whole. Indeed, Chelsea regretted having to engage in practices of self-care at all:

> I wish I could hand over my care to someone else and it would be like, "you sort out my health issues, you make me better in some way", and I don't feel that there is anyone I can hand it to, but that I have got to do all of that. I think that probably gets me down more than anything else because I would dearly love for this to be somebody else's responsibility, or at least to be able to trust someone else to make the right decisions and to be as invested as I am in getting me better or getting me to the point I want in my life. I think in that way that is really difficult, I think that there isn't that option. And that definitely makes me a lot tougher, but in some ways it also makes me a lot weaker because it takes up quite a large amount of mental and emotional and physical energy that you don't have for other things.

To the extent that Chelsea did engage with practices of self-care, like Alice and Yolanda, 'authenticity' was again a focus. When symptoms were at their worst, she almost felt as if she was watching herself 'becoming someone I am not really. So moody and quite aggressive and watching myself and hearing these things come out of my mouth, and just going *that is not me*, but I can't help it'. As she explained:

> I think I definitely used to just think something has to happen [in biomedical practice], because it can't be the way it is going to be, forever ... I think for a long time I felt that something can happen and it was all going to go away and that *I was going to go back to being that healthy person that I once was, somewhere a long time ago*. (my emphasis)

Here, Chelsea renders her pre-symptomatic self as 'healthy', thus positioning 'health' as a normative, preferable – and ultimately achievable – way of being. One function of this is to also position the experience of illness as inherently inauthentic and undesirable. I say this without wanting to discount the distressing aspects that are associated with the disease for a great number of women. Instead, my point is that self-care practices are at least partly understood as a method through which women might access a more valorised version of citizenship. To the extent that such a version of citizenship is symbolically adjacent to masculinity, then, I understand women's self-care practices as an attempt to disavow a devalued version of subjecthood that is assigned to them as endometriotic subjects, and to perform themselves as someone – or something – else altogether.

Empowerment and Agency

Although there are major differences between the accounts of Chelsea, Alice and Yolanda, all three women are attempting to rationalise and manage their *selves* following diagnosis. Alice and Yolanda perform themselves as initially naïve, confused, dysfunctional and disconnected from their bodies/selves, and later, as more connected, rational and responsible subjects. Chelsea's approach is more complicated, for although she resists medical formulations of herself as confused, dysfunctional and irrational, she does question the authenticity of her subjectivity and the extent to which she is capable of enacting a more stable and ordered subjecthood. In this sense, all three women's accounts exemplify the point, made earlier, that the actions women take after diagnosis are at least partially motivated by an attempt to construct oneself as rational, authentic and ordered. It is also difficult to know how to conceptualise the agency of these three women with respect to self-care. Although they are all 'enterprising' (Rose 1996) and pro-active, their activity stems from their exposure to and engagement with a range of ideas about women, menstruation and disease, including philosophies that suggest the roots of illness lay in the individual. Accordingly, women with endometriosis seem to understand endometriosis as a function of the diseased self. Self-care is also about trying to transcend the diseased self, which figures, paradoxically, as both a cause of the illness and an obstacle in the discovery of their authentic selves.

Are these practices, as others have suggested, 'empowering' for women? Undoubtedly, for some women, they are. Yolanda, for example, felt that taking more responsibility for her health had been beneficial:

> I think this was actually an empowering thing to do, taking an active role in my own health and wellbeing and resourcing how best to go about healing my symptoms. [It] helped me to access my own inner intuitive guidance and this has brought about many benefits in my life in general.

It is important to recognise the experience of responsibilisation as empowering, particularly for Alice and Yolanda. This is an important development, especially if women have previously felt powerless against a biomedical system that trivialised and dismissed their claims.[8] On the other hand, however, these accounts materialise a complex and complicated relationship to contemporary biomedicine, one in which women see themselves as, at times, overly medicalised, insufficiently medicalised, improperly medicalised, and compelled, in effect, to care for themselves. The fact that psychological explanations for the disease figure so heavily in all of the women's accounts is, I suggest, extremely significant. It is also unsurprising, to the extent that menstrual problems have traditionally figured as largely psychosomatic or psychogenic in both medical and self-help literature. For the same reasons, it is unsurprising to see women embarking upon an 'interior' search for answers and solutions regarding endometriosis. Whether this is ultimately positive or empowering, however, is doubtful.

Conclusion

In this chapter I have shown how an ethic of self-care emerges and figures in women's illness narratives, as well as the various ways this relates to understandings of self, body, rationality, authenticity, responsibility and citizenship. The range of practices with which women report engaging can be broadly defined, following Foucault, as technologies of the self. The state of 'happiness, purity, wisdom, perfection, or immortality' which women sought to attain included a desire to live a pain-free existence, to overcome illness, to get in touch with their authentic 'selves', and to become more rational. In relation to the latter, women recognised themselves as particular kinds of subjects – weak, disordered, and monstrous.

---

8   In this way, the women's experiences reflect those of other studies (e.g. Petersen 2006) in which individuals with health conditions have emphasised the positive aspects of their illness experience, including the positive aspects of becoming an 'expert' in their health.

The enactment of these subject positions can be described as part of a process of 'subjectification', which Nikolas Rose (1996: 11) defines as:

> Regimes of knowledge through which human beings have come to recognise themselves as certain kinds of creatures, the strategies of regulation and tactics of action to which these regimes of knowledge have been connected, and the correlative relations that human beings have established within themselves, in taking themselves as subjects.

Having recognised themselves as 'certain kinds of creatures', women utilised a range of technologies of the self – meditation, spiritual healing, counselling – in an attempt to manage and control those apparently problematic aspects of themselves. I have argued that these techniques are also gendered, in the sense that they simultaneously reflect and reproduce notions of femininity that are both familiar and concerning. One of the most striking aspects of women's narrative accounts is in the way the 'problem' requiring work is enacted. At first primarily concerned with menstrual pain and heavy bleeding – women came to see their dietary habits, lifestyle choices, exercise routines, emotional responses, coping mechanisms and very 'selves' as part of the overall problem requiring attention. This is important because, as I have earlier suggested, the management of women has long been a concern of medicine, especially gynaecological medicine.

Historically, medical experts have been central to this project, seeking to discover and correct the apparent secrets of women. Biomedicine has played an important role in the disciplining of women's bodies and in encouraging their compliance with the requirements of normative femininity, especially the need for women to be sexually and emotionally available to their partners and children and to fulfil their reproductive 'duties'. Now, by virtue of the way in which medicine is organised, applied, mediated, interpreted and lived in the present historical moment, the management of women is achieved not simply through the work of 'experts' (although they are, of course, involved); instead, it is achieved primarily through women's own 'entrepreneurship' (Rose 1996) – through governance of themselves. The fact that endometriosis is of uncertain aetiology is crucial to this expansionary project, because it allows exposure to an almost infinite number of ideas about the disease, its causation and management. In this respect, because almost anything might be a cause of the disease, virtually anything can become an object of scrutiny and self-management through practices of self-care.

The women I interviewed may be seeking to take 'charge', as the studies I quoted at the outset of this chapter suggested, but the important question is what they are seeking to take charge of. In my analysis, it is clear that women often seek to take charge of their monstrous bodies and disordered selves in ways that simultaneously reflect and reproduce normative ideas about gender. Applied to the present context, the sense of empowerment that may come from taking steps to manage one's own health is not merely the result of hopefulness that endometriosis symptoms may subside because of such action. Women are also relieved because they understand themselves to be moving closer towards, or enacting, a valorised form of subjecthood. They are, that is, behaving as rational, responsible citizens instead of maligned, indolent feminine subjects. These processes are extremely significant, politically and ethically, because even as women strive to exceed the confines of devalued feminine subjectivity that emerge in their narratives, they might reflect and reproduce those very same understandings of women: as 'passive', weak, irrational and sick. Self-care is thus a process via which women reproduce notions symbolically adjacent to the devalued 'feminine' and a method by which they attempt to transcend them. For many women this might just be an impossible paradox.

Women with endometriosis are positioned at the junction of two overlapping and contradictory versions of subjecthood. On the one hand, medicine constitutes them as less-than-full citizens: predominantly weak and irrational subjects in need of medical care and attention. On the other hand, women are constituted as rational and choosing subjects with the capacity to engage in forms of self-care. This dichotomous positioning amounts to something of a paradox for women and has parallels with some of my earlier work. In my research with Suzanne Fraser, for example (Fraser and Seear 2011; Seear and Fraser 2010a, 2010b), I have explored the challenges that many people who use drugs face in late, Western, discursive contexts. People positioned as drug 'addicts' are often constituted as chaotic subjects by virtue of their drug use, and are assumed to be incapable of making rational decisions. On the other hand, there is an increasing tendency to call upon people who inject drugs to engage in activities that are premised upon an understanding of them as rational, choosing and ordered subjects. For example, health promotion materials often call upon 'addicts' to avoid sharing toothbrushes, needles and ancillary injecting equipment. Here, 'addicts' are being enrolled into a wider public health strategy designed to reduce the rate of new infections for hepatitis C and other blood borne viruses. In this sense, then, people who inject drugs are simultaneously constituted as rational, choosing, irrational and disordered. There are several reasons why a dilemma like this might be of concern. Perhaps most obviously, this paradoxical positioning of 'addicts' raises major political questions, especially if public health campaigns to reduce the rate of new infections fail. Who, in those circumstances, is responsible? Is responsibility assigned back to the 'addict'? And to the extent it is, how might this function to reproduce them as disordered, irrational and irresponsible?

Although there are some parallels between that paradox and the one I have explored here, there are also a number of important differences. Most obviously, in the case of endometriosis, women are not subjected to the same kinds of stigmatising and marginalising discourses as are people who inject drugs. On the other hand, there are added layers of complexity and intrigue in the case of endometriosis, insofar as women are being encouraged to take action regarding an incurable disease of uncertain aetiology, where gendered psychological explanations of the disease figure centrally. The complexity of these issues is rendered apparent in the analysis of women's narratives that I have undertaken in this chapter. All of the women I interviewed engaged with psychological explanations of disease in some way following their diagnosis. This is a fraught practice, however, as the experiences of Chelsea demonstrate most clearly. Chelsea, we will recall, had lived with suspicions about her mental state for more than a decade. Although she vehemently resisted psychological prescriptions of her and her disease, she felt compelled, nevertheless, to engage in psychiatric treatment, partly as a way of demonstrating that she was not disordered. Ironically, Chelsea also recognised that the fact of her engagement with psychiatric medicine would now appear on her medical records for all time, and felt that this put her at risk of being labelled as unstable, disordered or irrational in the future. Although therapy is often understood as a form of self-care, there is a possibility that Chelsea's engagement with it produced her as the very kind of subject she was seeking to resist (recall, for instance, the way the sessions 'drove [her] nuts'). This demonstrates most vividly the almost impossible position that many women with endometriosis find themselves in following diagnosis, and the paradoxical implications of the way many of them engaged with self-care. Most often, women felt obliged to undertake emotional work, work on the self, or engage with psychological medicine or alternative medicine in ways that risked reproducing them as inherently disordered subjects. There is no easy way around all of this, of course, as Chelsea explicitly acknowledged. It seems that women with endometriosis must therefore try to negotiate a series of unenviable contradictions and paradoxes that are not of their making, nor of their choosing, in circumstances where few other options seem available to them. I recognise that this might appear to be a pessimistic reading. Nevertheless, I think it is important that we acknowledge these challenges, especially in light of previous accounts that have uncritically embraced women's 'responsibilising' turn. As the analysis in this chapter shows, a greater emphasis on 'self-care' does not necessarily mean that everything has now been put right for women with endometriosis, nor that gender is being made 'anew' in the process. There is some reason to be hopeful, however, as Annemarie Mol (2002) reminds us. As Mol (2002) points out, subjects and objects are not given in the order of things. Instead, of course, they materialise via practices, and to the extent that things are made in practice, through processes of constant iteration, things can always be made differently. I hope that this analysis might therefore signal the beginning of a more critical engagement with the way women are encouraged, in medicine, self-help and elsewhere, to engage with their disease following diagnosis so that we may consider new ways, little by little, to make things *anew*.

Conclusion:
Pinning Disease Down

That which is complex cannot be pinned down. To pin it down is to lose it.

(Mol and Law 2002: 21)

The becoming of the world is a deeply ethical matter.

(Barad 2007: 185)

I began this book with the short and seemingly simple question: *What is endometriosis?* This is a question that I have encountered many times over the last 20 years: as both a patient and a researcher. Each time it has been asked of me, or I have asked it, I have tended towards a different response, sometimes partial, sometimes more comprehensive, but always embedded in an appreciation of the considerable confusion and uncertainty associated with the disease. In this way, I have tended – largely unknowingly – towards an understanding of endometriosis as always already complex and messy, and as inherently changing and changeable. This is not, of course, how we are taught to think thought about ontology; indeed, my own way of thinking about endometriosis – indeed, about all objects and subjects – was originally one much more closely aligned with objectivist realism. If I had encountered this book at the start of my endometriosis journey, then, I may well have been frustrated by the approach that lay herein, insofar as the book offers no simple answers, preserves tensions and non-coherence, overlooks many practices associated with the disease, and makes no claims to completeness or to neatness. Mine is an account that is ultimately – necessarily – partial and messy. Although this may make for difficult reading, it is important, I suggest, not the least because it is faithful to the complexities and multiplicity of ontology.

Pinning Things Down

Preparing a conclusion for a book of this kind is therefore a challenge. What conclusions, if any, can be drawn? And what are the implications of eschewing a tidy finish? Might this produce yet another version of endometriosis – as fundamentally unstable and chaotic? (And would there be anything wrong with this, if so)? It would do to return to Annemarie Mol and John Law at this point, whose work has been so valuable in shaping my thinking throughout this book. In *Complexities* (2002: 21) Mol and Law argue that:

> Things add up *and* they don't. They flow in linear time *and* they don't. And they exist within a single space *and* escape from it. That which is complex cannot be pinned down. To pin it down is to lose it.

These insights certainly resonate with how I have understood (and performed) endometriosis in this book. There are things that flow and things that don't. There are things that add up and things that don't. So, for example, virtually all medical knowledge and practice is dominated by a faithful conviction to a single, fundamental and powerful idea: that endometriosis is a chronic gynaecological condition, connected to menstrual processes, peculiar to women. This is despite the evidence, noted in the Introduction, that endometriosis has been found in men's bodies, as well as in knees, lungs and brains. *So, things add up and they don't.* The point that Mol and Law are making, I think, is that we need not feel compelled to explain, negotiate or reconcile these apparent contradictions. Indeed, more might be gained from allowing these little curiosities to stand alongside one another, especially if we take the time to reflect on the possible wider significance of their presence (or absence, as the case may be) and how they are typically understood. How are these tensions handled? How, that is, do cases of endometriosis amongst men, and in knees, lungs and brains tend to be explained (if at all)? How do we produce these cases – as anomalies, mistakes, errors, or something else? What is being produced and reproduced as a consequence of these movements? What opportunities are made available? And what opportunities are lost?

As this simple example shows, I think, a refusal to navigate contradictions and resolve tensions can be productive: it may actually provoke new lines of inquiry about the politics and ethics of disease, and reveal the constitutive dimensions of assumptions, actions, movements. I also hope that my reluctance to produce a neat and 'definitive' account of the disease works as a reminder of the inherent challenges associated with trying to account for the complexity of the world, rather than an apparent admission of 'professional incompetence' (Mol and Law 2002: 7). If any conclusions *must* be drawn (and even that is not a given) then for what it is worth, I will offer this: endometriosis is an always already highly gendered, politicised phenomenon, the ontology of which is constant iteration. As well, articulations and practices pertaining to endometriosis work to leave behind 'traces' (Latour 2005) co-constituting, variously, gender, nature, culture, tradition and more, through intra-action with matter such as blood, tissue, treatment injunctions and drugs, theories of disease and more. In this way, the investigation I have undertaken in this book is one less concerned with trying to definitively capture the 'essence' of endometriosis than with exploring how disease and epidemic are being made, and what – in turn – disease and epidemic might be making. To some extent these intentions were signalled in the book's title, where I emphasised my desire to map some of the *makings* of the modern epidemic, *in this complex, multiple, performative sense*. I have not pinned the disease down, by any means, for to pin it down is to lose it, and – perhaps more importantly – to imply that our inquiries are at an end.

To say that I wanted to resist pinning endometriosis down is not to say that there are no observations that can be made about the disease. I want to turn, then, to some of the main observations this book sought to make about endometriosis, whilst simultaneously holding onto the idea, as far as that is possible, that my observations are inescapably partial and incomplete. The first point I made in this book is that endometriosis is not *just* a disease (as if there ever could be such a thing), but a complex political phenomenon. Or, to put this slightly differently, endometriosis is a phenomenon via which various norms are articulated, normative ideals produced and reproduced, and numerous 'threats' to the gendered, natural, human, traditional body are constituted (as I argued in Chapter 1). This reading of the disease/object has a range of implications for the subjects of the endometriosis epidemic, not the least of which was my point – made in the same chapter – that women with the disease figure as a symbolic and material hazard to be contained and controlled. Much of this book has been concerned with exploring how and where these acts of containment and control are occurring, as well as how and where these configurations might be challenged. One thread of this wider argument regarding the symbolic, material and political significance of the disease was that endometriosis figures as a 'crisis of the modern', an idea taken from two examples in medical activism where claims about the disease and its changing 'nature' have been made. To the extent that knowledges, practices and materialities pertaining to the disease are marked by flux, as I have argued, endometriosis also performs a remarkable continuity. As we head deeper into this century, then, it is crucial that we monitor how the disease continues to figure as crisis – symbolically, politically and materially – or not, so that we may develop a more nuanced and considered appreciation of why the disease matters, as well as the implications and 'effects' of these configurations for the subjects of this 'modern epidemic'.

In the second chapter, I examined a partially connected, partially disconnected phenomenon taking place within the medical literature. Focusing on the production, form and content of medical theories about the disease, I argued that medicine performs itself as heroic, progressive and omnipotent, while women and the feminine are performed as elusive, enigmatic and fundamentally disordered. In this sense, Chapter 2 introduced two of the key concerns of the book. First, it illustrated the productive dimensions of uncertainty, tension and debate within medical literature, arguing that although difference and uncertainty is a central feature of the medical literature, biomedicine regulates that difference and uncertainty in ways that preserve its own power. Secondly, I argued that medical literature is an exemplar of medicine's wider capacity to enact a set of hierarchical and necessarily problematic relations between itself and its subjects, and between subjects and disease. In focusing on the seemingly 'banal' phenomenon of disease theorisation, then, Chapter 2 also highlighted the political and ethical dimensions of disease theories for women living with endometriosis. Insofar as disease theories also produce and reproduce understandings of the 'normal' and 'natural' female body, the 'essence' of femininity, and more, they have, I argue, implications for women more broadly. The chapter also reminds us of the importance of examining discursive practices that may appear innocuous, unspectacular or far removed from ethics, politics and ontologies. Disease theories are always already all of these things (ethics, politics, and ontologies): far from banal, they are a set of thoroughly politicised processes for acting upon the world, enacting gender and distributing agency and power.

In Chapter 3, I examined a very different collection of texts: self-help books written for women living with the condition. I argued that self-help literature performs endometriosis as a largely coherent disease object, in contrast with the way the disease is enacted within some of the medical literature examined in Chapter 2. Self-help literature also preserves and performs a central contradiction of its own, however, by positioning the disease as simultaneously mysterious and uncertain, as well as stable and capable of being mastered. In this sense, self-help literature both reflects and reproduces a set of tensions that punctuate the field more broadly. Importantly, however, the way self-help literature 'handles' endometriosis (in the sense of approaching, and, in turn, enacting it) differs from other forms of textual 'representation' or articulation. Self-help literature has its own unique history, concerns and style, and thus enacts a version of the disease that overlaps with but also departs from the one we see within biomedical literature. In this sense, following Mol (2002), endometriosis emerges as 'more than one but less than many'. Arguing that these books also distribute agency in ways that are inherently problematic, I called for a more careful and considered approach to articulations of disease, agency and responsibility within self-help literature. One way this might be done is through a reappraisal of women's capacity for autonomous action, especially because, as I argued, injunctions to women are often offered with little or no consideration for how these configurations might mesh with women's lived experience of the disease.

Chapter 4 involved another reconsideration of medical knowledge and practice, this time through interviews with women who had been diagnosed with the disease. The focus was upon the connection between a central idea in endometriosis medicine – that the disease affects women who pertain to a 'typical patient profile' – and one aspect of medical practice: treatment. In that chapter, I challenged conventional understandings about the 'purpose', 'nature' and 'effects' of medical treatment, and of the way the subject figures in treatment, by arguing that medicine actually produces the very kinds of subject that it purports to merely be treating. This is a crucial idea, mainly because the 'typical patient profile' is central to endometriosis medical knowledge and practice, and, in many respects, to understandings about how the epidemic 'develops'. In this regard, Chapter 4 performs a reversal of its own, through disrupting taken-for-granted notions about cause and effect within disease populations. I concluded the chapter with a few suggestions about how treatment practices might be reconsidered, arguing that future practice should be guided – whatever the case – by the voices and experiences of women themselves. In a broader sense, this analysis also calls into question assumptions about what the epidemic 'is' and why the number of women being diagnosed with the condition is on the rise.

There is an important parallel to be drawn here, I want to suggest, between what is going on in endometriosis medicine and early (naïve) understandings of the HIV/AIDS epidemic: an idea, it will be recalled, that I explored at the outset of this book. In the introductory chapter I argued that in the initial stages of the HIV/AIDS epidemic, medical thought and practice was guided by a set of problematic assumptions about the subjects of disease and, by extension, cause and effect. Insofar as gay men were thought to be inherently (perhaps even 'naturally') promiscuous, contaminated and prone to risk-taking, and insofar as the disease was thought to be spread through sexual practices, a set of propositions about cause and effect emerged, took hold, and – a bit like a virus – spread. Other kinds of bodies were excluded from view, and with them, other possibilities for knowing the epidemic and intervening in its materiality. A similar phenomenon, I want to suggest, is to be found in operation here. Endometriosis medicine and practice has long been beholden to the notion that the endometriotic subject pre-exists her enrolment within medical practice, knowledge and discourse; alongside this, biomedicine has held steadfast to a set of beliefs about cause and effect – the vast majority of which rest upon assumptions about the subject's inherent 'nature', attitude, traits and so on. These ideas demand challenge, not in the least because they appear to be wrong, productive of stigma and marginalising in their effects, but also because they operate to obscure from view other possible – indeed, more plausible – explanations for the development and/or spread of the disease. In this sense, Chapter 4 touches upon one of the most important ideas in the book: that 'what is being made present always depends on what is also being made absent' (Law 2004: 83), both literally and metaphorically.

Although I would like to be in a position to extend these observations further, perhaps by making my own assertions about cause and effect, I understand that there are also dangers in doing so. And so, instead, I will offer some gestures and provocations, in the hope that these will generate further thinking and more research. At the very least, there is a need for a more critical and considered approach to the (largely crude, one-dimensional) way cause and effect is thought about in relation to the disease. We simply cannot persist with placing the endometriotic subject at the centre of accounts about cause and effect, while other agents – including medicine – are moved to the periphery. Strangely, perhaps, we see a focus on the agency and responsibility of women continuing to hold even as new ideas about the disease (like environmental theories) emerge. In this respect, we need to ask questions about the role that *all* subjects and objects might have in the manifestation of the nascent epidemic, including – crucially – medicine, doctors and scientists themselves. (I am thinking here about the diagnostic delay, and the role that medicine might play in shaping the materiality of the epidemic in at least this one respect). These questions can and should be extended to all of the 'actors' involved in the intra-active constitution of endometriosis as phenomenon. It would not do, as Callon and Latour (1997: 168) remind us, to 'bracket off' some 'things', or to persist with simplistic assumptions about agency, cause and effect. New ways of thinking through the epidemic are needed.

Finally, Chapter 5 examined a series of additional questions about how women engage with ideas about the disease and 'self-care' and with broader aspects of living with the condition. I argued that women's accounts of endometriosis were dominated by a sense of themselves as inherently dysfunctional, irrational and disordered, ideas closely associated with notions of menstruation and the feminine as monstrous. At the heart of women's lived experience with endometriosis is a central paradox: one where they feel obliged to correct problematic aspects of their self/body, but where doing so invariably reproduces them as devalued feminine subjects. The chapter concludes on an ambiguous and ambivalent note, questioning the utility of self-care arrangements for some women. To the extent that injunctions towards self-care can be found across multiple realms, which include – but are not limited to – self-help books and medical practice, there is a need to critically examine these for problematic and gendered depictions of menstruation, blood, female bodies, rationality, emotions and more. To the degree that these ideas and practices might also be tied to assumptions about how the disease is 'caused' and/or how it progresses, there is additional reason for concern, but also a space within which to ask extra questions about the various ways in which material-discursive formations may intra-actively co-constitute endometriosis as epidemic. To reiterate: this is not to question the existence (or otherwise) of the epidemic, in the same sense that critical approaches to the HIV/AIDS epidemic do not necessarily call into question the materiality of the disease or the realities of people who are living with AIDS. This approach to epidemics differs from an orthodox realist approach to science and medicine which sees the *epidemic as end game*: as an 'effect' or 'consequence' of either (or both) of the disease's 'natural' course and trajectory; and the behaviour/traits of (some – and only some) subjects in causing or contributing to these disease patterns. We would do well to take more seriously the implications of claims such as these, and commit to asking new and different questions about causality in which all manner of practices are understood as being implicated in the production of the world.

Back to the (Drawing) Board

One of the main inspirations for this study has been John Law's *Aircraft Stories* (2002), a text I have referred to throughout this book. Law describes that book as being:

> About specific episodes in a British attempt to build a military aircraft, a tactical strike and reconnaissance airplane, called the TSR2. (2002: 1)

He then explains that although:

> All the stories in the book are indeed about the TSR2, the book is really about something much more general. It is about modernism and its child,

postmodernism – and about how we might think past the limits these set to our ways of thinking. (2002: 1)

Law makes the point, which has of course been made elsewhere, that modernism and postmodernism are both problematic in their own respects; the former characterised by the 'homogeneities of centred storytelling' and the latter by 'pluralism of fragmentation'. His book constitutes an attempt to evade a choice between the two through what he calls 'fractional coherence' – the process, that is, of 'drawing things together without centring them' (2002: 2). In this book, I have tried to draw together various 'things' – textual and interview accounts of endometriosis, material-discursive practices across space and time – but without centering anything, through preserving the multiplicity of endometriosis as both a disease 'object' and political phenomenon, and by attending to some of the ways that endometriosis coheres – and does not – across space and time. The examples I explored in Chapter 1 exemplify this process, through illustrating some of the overlaps in understandings of what endometriosis 'is' across time, as well as the variation and variance therein. These observations might be extended, no doubt, to other spaces and places where endometriosis is materialised in local and specific forms – where 'patterns' of the disease diverge, and where understandings of menstruation, menstrual blood, fertility, reproductive potential and obligations differ, for instance, between cultures. In preserving these nuances, I hope to also provoke interest in the possibilities that exist to intervene in the making of the disease across space/time, in ways that will be ultimately less responsibilising, stigmatising and marginalising for women living with this complex, messy and poorly understood disease.

And so, with all of this in mind, I would like to reflect upon some of the key contributions, as I understand them, that this book seeks to make. I prefer to think of this list as a series of 'post-it' notes – if you can imagine them – arranged on a pinboard, none of which are any more important, meaningful or consequential than the next, but all of which, I hope, tell us something about the disease:

1. Endometriosis (and patterns pertaining to the disease) does not pre-exist 'social relations';
2. The ontology of objects and subjects are both 'enacted' and 'multiple', following Mol (2002);
3. The endometriotic subject does not pre-exist 'social relations';
4. Taken-for-granted ideas about the relationship between subjects, medicine and disease need to be revised, especially where those ideas produce problematic notions of cause and effect;
5. Complexity, instability, uncertainty and mess are productive;
6. All forms of articulation pertaining to endometriosis – including the ones I have examined here – but also others not covered in this book – operate to constitute the disease;

7. Following on from the above, we must attend to all forms – and forums – of articulation. Academic writing is not immune from this, and we must be 'equally' attentive to these issues;
8. Insofar as the ontology of endometriosis is constant iteration, there are always opportunities for the disease (and its subjects) to be made anew.

There are many more observations that might be made about endometriosis, and many more questions that need to be asked about the disease. And so this brings me to the end. Where, I ask, might we go from here?

Where to from Here?

Endometriosis is a disease marked by a curious duality. On the one hand, women are highly visible in endometriosis medicine. They are constituted as objects of both horror and fascination, as the likely source of the disease and thus an object to be measured, managed and mastered. Despite their ostensible visibility, however, women are also invisible in many important respects. In medical texts, journal articles and conference papers, physicians frequently talk *about* women without talking *to* them. There is virtually nothing of women's own voices in the historical canon: we do not know enough about how women experience diagnosis, life with the disease, and treatment. As we stand at the beginning of this century, we have a unique opportunity, as researchers, academics, patients, carers, family and friends, to pause and reflect upon how we want to deal with this duality. In this book, I have attempted to argue – with varying degrees of success, no doubt – that the way we manage, treat and practice disease is fundamentally connected to politics, ethics and ontology, with sometimes devastating implications for subjects. The traditional neglect of women's narratives has likely compounded these problems. As we consider where we might go from here, and what the analysis in this book offers us, it would do well to remind ourselves that nothing about this 'modern epidemic' amongst women should be taken for granted: not its form, 'effects', materiality, or 'nature'. Each of these things is shaped by and within the 'social' and, in turn, has the power to shape it. As we move forward, then, where might our priorities lie? What can be done? What might we hope to see five, 10, 50 or 100 years from now?

At the very least, I hope we will see more careful, considered and caring responses to women living with endometriosis, grounded, to a large extent, in the experiences of women themselves. Some of the biggest problems we face, as I see them, lay in the tendency to produce and reproduce women with the disease as simultaneously responsive and responsible, passive and agentive, in ways that almost always function to the detriment of the disease cohort. There is an incredible dearth of research that engages with these complexities and tensions, and although my work has attempted to correct some of these oversights there are many more issues that need to be considered. As well as this, new and purportedly more 'sophisticated' methods of diagnosis lay on the horizon, and different treatment modalities are being introduced, refined, and administered. We need to engage with the specific and local dimensions of these diagnostic techniques and treatment modalities, grounded, I suggest, in the voices of women themselves. How do women experience medical diagnosis, care and treatment? What new versions of self/body/agency are performed therein? Where are there inconsistencies and tensions in medical knowledge and practice, and how are they managed? How might we attend to absences and presences of the kind I described earlier in this chapter? For those of us who are interested in moving the research agenda forward, these represent a few ideas about where to start. There will, no doubt, be others.

This book has explored and inevitably *enacted* a series of connections and disconnections between different realms (in both space and time) where endometriosis is being/has been constituted. A critical study of the disease was vital, I suggested, because material-discursive practices cannot be separated out from questions about the constitution and distribution of agency, subjectivity, rights and responsibilities, and so, by extension, ethics, politics and power. As well as this, the study of endometriosis has helped us to 'trace' (Latour 2005) connections and associations in a series of small but significant ways, telling us something about the way disease participates in the making of the world (and of what is often referred to, uncritically, as 'the social'). This book has been concerned to demonstrate how health and illness can be understood *as politics* but without – and this is crucial – making any claim to be a complete account of those politics. These are serious questions, as Karen Barad reminds us, for they concern the becoming of the world, and '*the becoming of the world is a deeply ethical matter*' (2007: 185; my emphasis). I hope that the approach I have undertaken in this book may help to generate new insights into the relationship between diseases, subjects and epidemics – even if questions remain – and encourage a more careful approach to this grossly neglected disease. This was never going to be a complete or neutral analysis of the makings of this modern epidemic (indeed, it never could be). It was always a *view from somewhere*. But because we always have to start somewhere, I hope that this book will be taken for what it is: the beginning of a critical conversation about endometriosis, rather than the end of one.

Bibliography

Abbott, J.A., Hawe, J., Clayton, R.D. and Garry, R. 2003. The effects and effectiveness of laparoscopic excision of endometriosis: A prospective study with 2–5 year follow-up. *Human Reproduction*, 189, 1922–7.

Adkins, L. 2002. Reflexivity and the politics of qualitative research, in *Qualitative Research in Action*, edited by T. May. London: Sage, 332–48.

Agarwal, N. and Subramanian, A. 2010. Endometriosis – Morphology, Clinical Presentations and Molecular Pathology. *Journal of Laboratory Physicians*, 2(1), 1–9.

Ahmed, S. 2004a. Collective feelings, or the impressions left by others. *Theory, Culture and Society*, 21(2), 25–42.

Ahmed, S. 2004b. *The Cultural Politics of Emotion*. Edinburgh: Edinburgh University Press.

Altman, D. 1986. *AIDS and the New Puritanism*. Sydney: Pluto Press.

Altman, D. 1992. The most political of diseases, in *AIDS in Australia*, edited by E. Timewell, V. Minichiello and D. Plummer. Sydney: Prentice Hall.

American Endometriosis Association 2009. *Endometriosis and Dioxins: Information for Physicians, Nurses, and Other Health Care Professionals.* Wisconsin: Endometriosis Association.

Armstrong, D. 1984. The patient's view. *Social Science and Medicine*, 18, 737–44.

Arruda, M.S., Petta, C.A., Abrao, M.S and Benetti-Pinto, C.L. 2003. Time elapsed from onset of symptoms to diagnosis of endometriosis in a cohort study of Brazilian women. *Human Reproduction*, 184, 756–9.

Atthill, L. 1883. *Clinical Lectures on Diseases Peculiar to Women.* 7th Edition. Dublin: Fannin and Co.

Bacchi, C.L. and C. Beasley 2002. Citizen bodies: is embodied citizenship a contradiction in terms? *Critical Social Policy*, 22(2), 324–52.

Ballard, K., Lowton, K. and Wright, J. 2006. What's the delay? A qualitative study of women's experiences in reaching a diagnosis of endometriosis. *Fertility and Sterility*, 86(5), 1296–301.

Ballweg, M.L. 1992. Endometriosis: The patient's perspective. *Infertility and Reproductive Medicine Clinics of North America*, 3(3), 747–61.

Ballweg, M.L. 1997. Blaming the victim: The psychologizing of endometriosis. *Obstetrics and Gynecology Clinics of North America*, 24(2), 441–53.

Ballweg, M.L. 2003a. Research reveals disease is starting younger, diagnosis is delayed, in *Endometriosis: The Complete Reference for Taking Charge of Your Health,* edited by M.L. Ballweg and the Endometriosis Association. Chicago, USA: Contemporary Books, 343–60.

Ballweg, M.L. 2003b. Endometriosis walk for awareness: Our movement goes public, in *Endometriosis: The Complete Reference for Taking Charge of Your Health*, edited by M.L. Ballweg and the Endometriosis Association. United States of America: Contemporary Books, 375–7.

Ballweg, M.L. 2003c. Preventing endometriosis: It may be possible! in *Endometriosis: The Complete Reference for Taking Charge of Your Health*, edited by M.L. Ballweg and the Endometriosis Association. United States of America: Contemporary Books, 305–40.

Ballweg, M.L. 2003d. What is Endometriosis?, in *Endometriosis: The Complete Reference for Taking Charge of Your Health*, edited by M.L. Ballweg and the Endometriosis Association. United States of America: Contemporary Books, 1–6.

Ballweg, M.L. 2003e. Joe with Endo, in *Endometriosis: The Complete Reference for Taking Charge of Your Health*, edited by M.L. Ballweg and the Endometriosis Association. United States of America: Contemporary Books, 381–406.

Ballweg, M.L. 2003f. Impact of endometriosis on women's health: Comparative historical data show that the earlier the onset, the more severe the disease. *Best Practice and Research Clinical Obstetrics and Gynaecology*, 18(2), 201–18.

Ballweg, M.L. and the Endometriosis Association 2003. *Endometriosis: The Complete Reference for Taking Charge of Your Health*. Chicago, USA: Contemporary Books.

Barad, K. 1998. Getting real: Technoscientific practices and the materialization of reality. *Differences: A Journal of Feminist Cultural Studies*, 10(2), 87–128.

Barad, K. 2003. Posthumanist performativity: Toward an understanding of how matter comes to matter. *Signs: Journal of Women in Culture and Society*, 28(3), 801–31.

Barad, K. 2007. *Meeting the Universe Halfway: Quantum Physics and the Entanglement of Matter and Meaning*. Durham: Duke University Press.

Barnard A. 2001. Endometriosis and pain, in *Pain in Obstetrics and Gynaecology*, edited by A.B. McClean, R.W. Stones and S. Thornton. London: Royal College of Obstetrics and Gynaecology Press, 145–51.

Batt, R. 2011. *A History of Endometriosis*. London and New York: Springer.

Bauman, Z. 2000. *Liquid Modernity*. Cambridge: Polity Press.

Beck, U. 1992. *Risk Society: Towards a New Modernity*. London: Sage.

Beckman, E.N., Pintado, S.O., Leonard, G.L. and Sternberg, W.H. 1985. Endometriosis of the prostate. *American Journal of Surgical Pathology*, 9(5), 374–9.

Benagiano, G. and Brosens, I. 1991. The history of endometriosis: identifying the disease. *Human Reproduction*, 6(7), 963–8.

Benagiano, G. and Brosens, I. 2006. History of adenomyosis, *Best Practice and Research Clinical Obstetrics and Gynaecology*, 20(4), 449–63.

Berbic, M. and Fraser, I.S. 2011. Regulatory T cells and other leukocytes in the pathogenesis of endometriosis. *Journal of Reproductive Immunology*, 88(2), 149–55.

Berger, P. and Luckmann, T. 1966. *The Social Construction of Reality: A Treatise in the Sociology of Knowledge*. Harmondsworth, Middlesex: Penguin Books.

Birnbaum, L. and Cummings, A. 2002. Endometriosis and dioxins: A plausible hypothesis. *Environmental Health Perspectives*, 110(1), 15–21.

Bland-Sutton, J. and Giles, A. 1916. *The Diseases of Women: A Handbook for Students and Practitioners*. 7th Edition. London: William Heinemann.

Bodner, C., Garratt, A.M., Ratcliffe, J., et al. 1997. Measuring health-related quality of life outcomes in women with endometriosis: Results of the gynaecology audit project in Scotland. *Health Bulletin (Edinburgh)*, 55, 109–17

Boling, R.O., Abbasi, R., Ackerman, G., Schipul, A. and Chaney, S. 1988. Disability from endometriosis in the United States army. *Journal of Reproductive Medicine*, 33, 1, 49–52.

Boston Women's Health Book Collective 1973. *Our Bodies, Ourselves*. New York: Simon and Schuster.

Boston Women's Health Book Collective 1984. *The New Our Bodies, Ourselves: A Book by and for Women*. New York: Simon and Schuster.

Braidotti, R. 1994. *Nomadic Subjects: Embodiment and Sexual Difference in Contemporary Feminist Theory*. New York: Columbia University Press.

Brewer, S. 1995. *Endometriosis and Fibroids: The Complete Guide to the Causes, the Symptoms and the Treatments*. London: Vermilion

Brosens, I.A. and Brosens, J.J. 2000. Review: Endometriosis. *European Journal of Obstetrics and Gynecology and Reproductive Biology*, 90, 159–64.

Buck Louis, G.M., Weiner, J.M., Whitcomb, B.W., et al. 2005. Environmental PCB exposure and risk of endometriosis. *Human Reproduction*, 20(1), 279–85.

Bunton, R. and Burrows, R. 1995. Consumption and Health in the 'epidemiological' clinic of late modern medicine, in *The Sociology of Health Promotion: Critical Analyses of Consumption, Lifestyle and Risk*, edited by R. Bunton, S. Nettleton and R. Burrows. London: Routledge, 206–22.

Burchell, G. 1996. Liberal government and techniques of the self, in *Foucault and Political Reason: Liberalism, Neo-Liberalism and Rationalities of Government*, edited by A. Barry, T. Osborne and N. Rose. Chicago: University of Chicago Press, 19–36.

Bury, M. 1997. *Health and Illness in a Changing Society*. London: Routledge.

Butler, J. 1990. *Gender Trouble: Feminism and the Subversion of Identity*. New York: Routledge.

Butler, J. 1993. *Bodies That Matter: On the Discursive Limits of 'Sex'*. New York: Routledge.

Callahan, T.L., Caughey, A.B. and Heffner, L. 2004. *Blueprints: Obstetrics and Gynecology*. 3rd Edition. Massachusetts: Blackwell Publishing.

Callon, M. 1986. Some elements of a sociology of translation: Domestication of the scallops and the fishermen of St. Brieuc Bay, in *Power, Action and Belief:*

A New Sociology of Knowledge?, edited by J. Law. London: Routledge and Kegan Paul, 196–233.

Callon, M. 1999. Actor-network theory: the market test, in *Actor Network Theory and After*, edited by J. Law and J. Hassard. Oxford: Blackwell Publishing, 181–95.

Callon, M. and Latour, B. 1992. Don't throw the baby out with the Bath school! in *Science As Practice and Culture*, edited by A. Pickering. Chicago: University of Chicago Press, 343–68.

Callon, M. and Law, J. 1997. After the Individual in Society: Lessons on collectivity from science, technology and society. *Canadian Journal of Sociology*, 22(2), 165–82.

Campbell, J.S., Wong, J., Tryphonas, L., et al. 1985. Is simian endometriosis an effect of immunotoxicity? Presented at the Ontario Association of Pathologists 48th Annual Meeting, London, Ontario.

Carlton, D. 1996. Awareness of endometriosis. *Practice Nurse*, 12, 514–15.

Carpan, C. 2003. Representations of endometriosis in the popular press: 'The career woman's disease'. *Atlantis*, 27(2), 1–15.

Carter, K.C. 2003. *The Rise of Causal Concepts of Disease: Case Histories.* Aldershot: Ashgate.

Capek, S. 2000. Reframing endometriosis: From 'career woman's disease' to environment/body Connections, in *Illness and the Environment: A Reader in Contested Medicine*, edited by S. Kroll-Smith, P. Brown and V.J. Gunter. New York: New York University Press, 345–63.

Casper, M. 1994. Reframing and grounding nonhuman agency: What makes a fetus an agent? *American Behavioral Scientist*, 37(6), 839–56.

Castel, R. 1991. From dangerousness to risk, in *The Foucault Effect: Studies in Governmentality*, edited by G. Burchell, C. Gordon. and P. Miller. Brighton: Harvester Wheatsheaf, 281–98.

Chalmers, J.A. 1975. *Endometriosis*. London: Butterworths.

Chandler, J. 2000. Endometriosis: The disease of theories. *Postgraduate Medicine*, 107, 213–24.

Charmaz, K. 1983. Loss of self: A fundamental form of suffering in the chronically ill. *Sociology of Health and Illness*, 5, 168–95.

Cheek, J. and Rudge, T. 1997. The rhetoric of health care? Foucault, health care practices and the docile body – 1990s style, in: *Foucault: The Legacy*, edited by C. O'Farrell. Kelvin Grove: Queensland University of Technology, 707–13.

Churchill, F. 1885. *Outlines of the Principal Diseases of Females: Chiefly for the Use of Students*. Dublin: Martin Keene and Son.

Colborn, T., Dumanoski, D. and Myers, J.P. 1997. *Our Stolen Future: Are We Threatening Our Fertility, Intelligence, and Survival? – A Scientific Detective Story*. London: Abacus.

Collins, H. and Yearley, S. 1992. Epistemological chicken, in *Science as Practice and Culture*, edited by A. Pickering. Chicago: University of Chicago Press, 301–26.

Cooke, K. and Trickey, R. 2002. *Endometriosis: Natural and Medical Solutions*. Crows Nest: Allen and Unwin.

Cox, H., Henderson, L., Anderson, N., et al. 2003b. Focus group study of endometriosis: Struggle, loss and the medical merry-go-round. *International Journal of Nursing Practice*, 9, 2–9.

Cox, H., Henderson, L., Wood, R. and Cagliarini, G. 2003c. Learning to take charge: women's experiences of living with endometriosis', *Complementary Therapies in Nursing and Midwifery*, 9, 62–8.

Cox, H., Ski, C.F., Wood, R., and Sheahan, M. 2003a. Endometriosis; an unknown entity: the consumer's perspective. *International Journal of Consumer Studies*, 27(3), 200–209.

Crawford, R. 1980. Healthism and the medicalization of everyday life. *International Journal of Health Services*, 10(3), 365–88.

Creed, B. 2007. *The Monstrous-Feminine: Film, Feminism, Psychoanalysis*. New York: Routledge.

Daykin, N. and Naidoo, J. 1995. Feminist critiques of health promotion, in *The Sociology of Health Promotion: Critical Analyses of Consumption, Lifestyle and Risk*, edited by R. Bunton, S. Nettleton and R. Burrows. London: Routledge, 59–69.

Deleuze, G. 1994. *Difference and Repetition*. London: Athlone Press.

Denny, E. 2004a. Women's experience of endometriosis. *Journal of Advanced Nursing*, 46(6), 641–8.

Denny, E. 2004b. 'You are one of the unlucky ones': Delay in the diagnosis of Endometriosis. *Diversity in Health and Social Care*, 1, 39–44.

Denny, E. and Khan, S. 2006. Systematic reviews of qualitative evidence: What are the experiences of women with endometriosis? *Journal of Obstetrics and Gynaecology*, 26(6), 501–6.

Denny, E. and Mann, C. 2007. Endometriosis-associated dyspareunia: the impact on women's lives. *Journal of Family Planning and Reproductive Health Care*, 33(3), 189–93.

Derrida, J. 1976. *Of Grammatology*. Baltimore: Johns Hopkins University Press. (Translated by G.C. Spivak.)

Derrida, J. 2002. *Writing and Difference*. London: Routledge. (Translated by A. Bass.)

Domar, A.D. and Dreher, H. 1996. *Healing Mind, Healthy Woman*. London: Thorsons.

Donnez, J., Nisolle, M. and Casanas-Roux, F. 1994. Peritoneal Endometriosis: two-dimensional and three-dimensional evaluation of typical and subtle lesions. *Annals of the New York Academy of Sciences*, 734, 342–51.

Dougherty, E. 2004. Options when endo makes it hard to get pregnant, in *Endometriosis: The Complete Reference for Taking Charge of Your Health*, edited by M.L. Ballweg and the Endometriosis Association. United States of America: Contemporary Books, 133–51.

Douglas, M. 1990. Risk as a forensic resource. *Daedalus*, Fall 1990, 1–16.

Duff, C.J. 2012. After methods, after subjects, after drugs. *Contemporary Drug Problems*, 39(2), 265–87.

Duff, C. 2013. The social life of drugs. *International Journal of Drug Policy*, Vol. 24, No. 3, 167–72.

Duffin, J. 2005. *Lovers and Livers: Disease Concepts in History.* Toronto: University of Toronto Press.

Dwyer, R. and Moore, D. 2013. Enacting multiple methamphetamines: The ontological politics of public discourse and consumer accounts of a drug and its effects. *International Journal of Drug Policy*, 24(3), 203–11.

Ehrenreich, B. and English, D. 1978. *For Her Own Good: 150 Years of the Experts' Advice to Women.* New York: Doubleday.

Ellingson, L. 2006. Embodied knowledge: Writing researchers' bodies into qualitative health research. *Qualitative Health Research*, 16(2), 298–310.

Emad. M. 2006. At WITSENDO: Communal embodiment through storytelling in women's experiences with endometriosis. *Women's Studies International Forum*, 29, 197–207.

Evans, S., 2005. *Endometriosis and Other Pelvic Pain*. South Melbourne: Thomas C. Lothian Pty Ltd.

Evers, J. 1994. Endometriosis does not exist; all women have endometriosis. *Human Reproduction*. 9(12), 2206–9.

Evers, J. 1996. The defense against endometriosis. *Fertility and Sterility*, 66(3), 351–3.

Evers, J. 2010. Introduction, in *Endometriosis: Current Management and Future Trends,* edited by J. Garcia-Velasco and B. Rizk. New Delhi: Jaypee, xvii–xviii.

Finlay, L. 1998. Reflexivity: An essential component for all research? *British Journal of Occupational Therapy*, 61, 453–6.

Finlay, L. 2002. 'Outing' the researcher: The provenance, process, and practice of reflexivity. *Qualitative Health Research*, 12(4), 531–45.

Foucault, M. 1977. *Discipline and Punish.* Harmondsworth: Penguin.

Foucault, M. 1978. *The History of Sexuality Volume 1: An Introduction.* New York: Random House.

Foucault, M. 1980a. Body/Power, in *Power/Knowledge: Selected Interviews and Other Writings 1972–1977,* edited by C. Gordon. New York: Random House, 55–62.

Foucault, M. 1980b. Two Lectures, in *Power/Knowledge: Selected Interviews and Other Writings 1972–1977,* edited by C. Gordon. New York: Random House, 78–108.

Foucault, M. 1980c. Power and Strategies, in *Power/Knowledge: Selected Interviews and Other Writings 1972–1977,* edited by C. Gordon. New York: Random House, 134–45.

Foucault, M. 1988. Technologies of the Self, in *Technologies of the Self: A Seminar with Michel Foucault*, edited by L.H. Martin, H. Gutman and P.H. Hutton. Amherst: The University of Massachusetts Press, 16–49.

Foucault, M. 2002. *The Archaeology of Knowledge.* London: Routledge.

Fraser, S. 2004. 'It's Your Life!': Injecting drug users, individual responsibility and hepatitis C prevention, *Health: An Interdisciplinary Journal for the Social Study of Health, Illness and Medicine*, 8(2), 199–221.

Fraser, S. 2006. The chronotope of the queue: Methadone maintenance treatment and the production of time, space and subjects. *International Journal of Drug Policy*, 17(13), 192–202.

Fraser, S. and Moore, D. 2011. *The Drug Effect: Health, Crime and Society*. Melbourne: Cambridge University Press.

Fraser, S. and Seear, K. 2011. *Making Disease, Making Citizens: The Politics of Hepatitis C*. Aldershot: Ashgate.

Freud, S. 1973. *New Introductory Lectures on Psycho-Analysis*. London: Penguin.

Friedson, E. 1970. *Profession of Medicine: A Study of the Sociology of Applied Knowledge*. New York: Dodd, Mead and Company.

Fukunaga, M. 2012. Paratesticular endometriosis in a man with a prolonged hormonal therapy for prostatic carcinoma. *Pathology Research and Practice*, 208(1), 59–61.

Fullagar, S. 2002. Governing the healthy body: discourses of leisure and lifestyle within Australian health policy. *Health: An Interdisciplinary Journal for the Social Study of Health, Illness and Medicine*, 61, 69–84.

Galvin, R. 2002. Disturbing notions of chronic illness and individual responsibility: towards a genealogy of morals. *Health: An Interdisciplinary Journal for the Social Study of Health, Illness and Medicine*, 6(2), 107–37.

Gao, X., Outley, J., Botteman, M., Spalding, J., et al. 2006. Economic burden of endometriosis. Fertility and Sterility, 86(6), 1561–72.

Garry, R., Clayton, R. and Hawe, J. 2000. The effect of endometriosis and its radical laparoscopic excision on quality of life indicators. *British Journal of Obstetrics and Gynaecology*, 107, 44–54.

Gerhard, I. and Runnebaum, B. 1992. Grenzen der Hormonsubstitution bei Schadstoffbelastung und Fertilitatsstorungen. Zentralbl Gynakol, 114, 593–602.

Giannarini, G., Scott, C.A., Moro, U., et al. 2006. Cystic endometriosis of the epididymis. *Urology*, 68(1), 203.e1–3.

Giddens, A. 1991. *Modernity and Self-Identity: Self and Society in the Late Modern Age*. Cambridge: Polity Press.

Giudice, L. 2010. Clinical practice: Endometriosis. *New England Journal of Medicine*, 362(25), 2389–98.

Giudice, L., Evers, J. and Healy, D. 2012. *Endometriosis: Science and Practice*. Chichester: Wiley Blackwell.

Giudice, L. and Kao, L. 2004. Endometriosis. *The Lancet*, 364(9447), 1789–99.

Goode, E. and Ben-Yehuda, N. 1994. Moral panics: Culture, politics and social construction. *Annual Review of Sociology*, 20, 149–71.

Green, M.S., Swartz, T., Mayshar, E., et al. 2002. When is an epidemic an epidemic? *Israel Medical Association Journal*, 4(1), 3–6.

Grodin, D. 1991. The interpreting audience: The therapeutics of self-help book reading. *Critical Studies in Mass Communication*, 8, 404–20.

Grosz, E.A. 1989. *Sexual Subversions: Three French Feminists*. Sydney: Allen and Unwin.

Grosz, E.A. 1994. *Volatile Bodies: Towards a Corporeal Feminism*. Indiana: Indiana University Press.

Guo, S. 2004. The link between exposure to dioxin and endometriosis: a critical reappraisal of primate data. *Gynecologic and Obstetric Investigation*, 57, 157–73.

Hacking, I. 1986. Making up people, in *Reconstructing Individualism: Autonomy, Individuality and the Self in Western Thought*, edited by T.C. Heller. Stanford, CA: Stanford University Press, 222–36.

Hacking, I. 1999. *The Social Construction of What?* Cambridge, Massachusetts: Harvard University Press.

Hadfield, R., Mardon, H., Barlow, D. and Kennedy, S. 1996. Delay in the diagnosis of endometriosis: a survey of women from the USA and the UK. *Human Reproduction*, 11(4), 878–80.

Hahn, R. 1995. *Sickness and Healing: An Anthropological Perspective*. New Haven: Yale University Press.

Haraway, D. 1985. A cyborg manifesto: Science, technology, and socialist-feminism in the late twentieth century. *Socialist Review*, 80, 65–108.

Haraway, D. 1991. *Simians, Cyborgs and Women: The Reinvention of Nature*. London: Free Association.

Harding, S. 1986. *The Science Question in Feminism*. Ithaca: Cornell University Press.

Harding, S. 1987. *Feminism and Methodology: Social Science Issues*. Indiana University Press: Bloomington.

Henderson, L. and Wood, R. 2000. *Explaining Endometriosis*. 2nd Edition. Crow's Nest: Allen and Unwin.

Hermann, G.E. 1899. *Diseases of Women: A Clinical Guide to Their Diagnosis and Treatment*. London: Cassell and Co.

Hochschild, A. 2003. *The Managed Heart: Commercialization of Human Feeling*. 2nd Edition. Berkeley: University of California Press.

Hochschild, A.R. 1994. The Commercial spirit of intimate life and the abduction of feminism: Signs from women's advice books. *Theory, Culture and Society*, 11, 1–24.

Holloway, M. 1994. An epidemic ignored. *Scientific American*, April, 24–7.

Hornstein, M.D., Surrey, E.S., Weisberg, G.W. and Casino, L.A. 1998. Leuprolide acetate depot and hormonal add-back in endometriosis: A 12–month study. *Obstetrics and Gynecology*, 91, 16–24.

Hughes, E. 1997. Health promotion and 'non-compliance' – an analysis of resistance to regulatory technologies. *Annual Review of Health Social Sciences*, 7, 18–27.

Husby, G.K., Haugen, R.S. and Moen, M.H. 2003. Diagnostic delay in women with pain and endometriosis. *Acta Obstetricia et Gynecologica Scandinavica*. 827, 649–53.

Illich, I. 1976. *Medical Nemesis*. New York: Pantheon Books.

Irigaray, L. 1985. *Speculum of the Other Woman.* USA: Cornell University Press. (Translated by G.C. Gill.)

Jaffe, R. 2004. Foreword, in *Endometriosis: The Complete Reference for Taking Charge of Your Health,* edited by M.L. Ballweg and the Endometriosis Association. United States of America: Contemporary Books, xv–xvii.

Jones, G., Kennedy, S., Barnard, A., et al. 2001. Development of an endometriosis Quality-of-Life instrument: The endometriosis health profile-30. *Obstetrics and Gynecology,* 98(2), 258–64.

Jones, K.B. 1998. Citizenship in a woman-friendly polity, in *The Citizenship Debates: A Reader,* edited by G. Shafir. Minneapolis: University of Minnesota Press, 221–47.

Kasperson, R.E., Renn, O., Slovic, P., et al. 1988. The social amplification of risk: a conceptual framework. *Risk Analysis,* 8(2), 177–87.

Kennedy. S. 2005. Who gets endometriosis? *Women's Health Medicine,* 2(1), 18–19.

Kennedy, S., Bergqvist, A., Chapron, C., et al. on behalf of the ESHRE Special Interest Group for Endometriosis and Endometrium Guideline Development Group 2005. ESHRE guideline for the diagnosis and treatment of endometriosis. *Human Reproduction,* 20(10), 2698–704.

Kiesel, L.A., Rody, A., Greb, R. and Szilagyi, A. 2002. Clinical use of GnRH analogues. *Clinical Endocrinology,* 56, 677–87.

Kirby, V. 2006. *Judith Butler: Live Theory.* London: Continuum.

Kistner, R.W. 1971. *Gynecology: Principles and Practice.* 2nd Edition. Chicago: Year Book Medical Publishers.

Kitzinger, J. 1999. Researching risk and the media. *Health, Risk and Society,* 1(1), 55–69.

Knapp, V.J. 1999. How old is endometriosis? Late 17th- and 18th-century European descriptions of the disease, *Fertility and Sterility,* 72(1), 10–14.

Koski, C.A. 1995. An epidemic ignored. *Chattanooga Free Press:* B1–B2 (May 23).

Kristeva, J. 1982. *Powers of Horror: An Essay on Abjection.* New York: Columbia University Press. (Translated by L.S. Roudiez.)

Kroger, W.S and Freed, S.C. 1962. *Psychosomatic Gynecology: Including Problems and Obstetrical Care.* California: Wilshire Book Company.

Krotec, J. and Perkins, S. 2007. *Endometriosis for Dummies.* Hoboken: Wiley Publishing.

Kumar, S., Tiwari, P., Sharma, P., et al. 2012. Urinary Tract Endometriosis: A Review of 19 cases. *Urology Annals,* 4(1), 6–12.

Latour, B. 1986. Visualisation and Cognition: Drawing things together, in *Knowledge and Society Studies in the Sociology of Culture Past and Present,* edited by H. Kuklick, 6, 1–40.

Latour, B. 1987. *Science in Action: How to Follow Scientists and Engineers Through Society.* Cambridge: Harvard University Press.

Latour, B. (as Jim Johnson). 1988a. Mixing humans and nonhumans together: The sociology of a door-closer. *Social Problems*, 35(3), Special Issue: The Sociology of Science and Technology. 298–310.

Latour, B. 1988b. How to write *The Prince* for machines as well as for machinations, in *Technology and Social Change*, edited by B. Elliot. Edinburgh: Edinburgh University Press, 20–63.

Latour, B. 2005. *Reassembling the Social: An Introduction to Actor-Network Theory*. New York: Oxford University Press.

Latour, B. and Woolgar, S. 1986. *Laboratory Life: The Social Construction of Scientific Facts*. Beverley Hills: Sage Publications.

Lauersen, N. and Whitney, S. 1977. *It's Your Body: A Woman's Guide to Gynaecology*. New York: Grosset and Dunlop.

Lauersen, N.H. and deSwann, C. 1988. *The Endometriosis Answer Book: New Hope, New Help*. New York: Rawson Associates.

Law, J. 1987. Technology and heterogeneous engineering: The case of Portuguese expansion, in *The Social Construction of Technological Systems*, edited by W.E. Bijker, T. Hughes and T. Pinch. Cambridge: MIT Press, 111–34.

Law, J. 1994. *Organizing Modernity: Social Ordering and Social Theory*. Oxford: Blackwell Publishers.

Law, J. 1999. After ANT: complexity, naming and topology, in *Actor Network Theory and After*, edited by J. Law and J. Hassard. Oxford: Blackwell, 1–14.

Law, J. 2002. *Aircraft Stories: Decentering the Object in Technoscience*. Durham: Duke University.

Law, J. 2004. *After Method: Mess in Social Science Research*. London and New York: Routledge.

Law, J. 2007. Pinboards and books: Learning, materiality and juxtaposition, in *Education and Technology: Critical Perspectives, Possible Futures*, edited by D. Kritt and L. Winegar. Lanham, Maryland. Lexington Books, 125–50.

Lebel, G., Dodin, S., Ayotte, P., et al. 1998. Organochloride exposure and the risk of endometriosis. *Fertility and Sterility*, 69(2), 221–8.

Letherby, G. 2003. *Feminist Research in Theory and Practice*. Buckingham: Open University Press.

Levett, C. 2008. *Reclaim Your Life: Your Guide to Aid Healing of Endometriosis*.

Lewis, D.O., Comite, F., Mallouh, C., et al. 1987. Bipolar Mood Disorder and Endometriosis: Preliminary Findings. *American Journal of Psychiatry*, 144(12), 1588–91.

Lupton, D. 1993. AIDS risk and heterosexuality in the Australian press. *Discourse and Society*, 4(3), 307–28.

Lupton, D. 1997. Foucault and the Medicalisation Critique, *Foucault, Medicine and Health*, edited by A. Petersen and R. Bunton. London: Routledge, 94–110.

Lupton, D. 2003. *Medicine as Culture*. 2nd Edition. London: Sage.

Lupton, D. 2004. 'A grim health future': food risks in the Sydney press. *Health, Risk and Society*, 6(2), 187–200.

Lupton, D. 2005. Risk as moral danger: the social and political functions of risk discourse in public health, in: *The Sociology of Health and Illness: Critical Perspectives*, edited by P. Conrad. New York: Worth Publishers, 422–9.

Lyons, A. and Griffin, C. 2003. Managing menopause: a qualitative analysis of self-help literature for women at midlife. *Social Science and Medicine*, 56, 1629–42.

Lyons, T. and Kimball, C. 2003. *What to Do When the Doctor Says It's Endometriosis*. Gloucester, MA: Fair Winds Press.

Magdalinski, T. 2009. *Sport, Technology and the Body: The Nature of Performance* Abingdon, Oxon: Routledge.

Makita, K., Ishitana, K., Ohta, H., et al. 2005. Long-term effects on bone mineral density and bone metabolism of 6 months' treatment with gonadotropin-releasing hormone analogues in Japanese women: comparison of buserelin acetate with leuprolide acetate. *Journal of Bone and Mineral Metabolism*, 23, 389–94.

Manderson, L., Warren, N. and Markovic, M. 2008. Circuit breaking: Pathways of treatment seeking for women with endometriosis in Australia. *Qualitative Health Research*, 18(4), 522–34.

Mantel, H. 2003. *Giving Up the Ghost: A Memoir.* New York: Picador.

March, J. 1994. *A Primer On Decision Making: How Decisions Happen.* New York: The Free Press.

Marshall, C. and Rossman, G. 1989. *Designing Qualitative Research.* Newbury Park, CA: Sage.

Martin, E. 1987. *The Woman in the Body: A Cultural Analysis of Reproduction.* 2nd Edition. Boston: Beacon Press.

Martin, J.D. and Hauck, A.E. 1985. Endometriosis in the male. *The American Surgeon*, 51(7), 426–30.

Martin, K. 2003. Giving birth like a girl. *Gender and Society*, 17(1), 54–72.

Mayani, A., Barel, S., Soback, S. and Almagor, M. 1997. Dioxin concentrations in women with endometriosis. *Human Reproduction*, 12(2), 373–5.

Mears, J. 1996. *Coping with Endometriosis*. London: Sheldon Press.

Meigs, J.V. 1938. Editorial: Endometriosis – A possible etiologic factor. *Surgery, Gynecology and Obstetrics*, 67.

Meigs, J.V. 1941. Endometriosis – Its significance. *Annals of Surgery*, 114(5), 866–74.

Meigs, J.V. 1948. Endometriosis. *Annals of Surgery*, 127(5), 795–808.

Meigs, J.V. 1950. Discussion. *Annals of Surgery*, 131(5), 719.

Meigs, J.V. 1953. Endometriosis: Etiologic role of marriage age and parity; conservative treatment. *Obstetrics and Gynecology*, 2(1), 46–53.

Mills, D.S. and Vernon, M. 2002. *Endometriosis: A Key to Healing Through Nutrition*. London: Thorsens.

Missmer, S.A and Cramer, D.W. 2003. Epidemiology of endometriosis. *Obstetrics and Gynecology Clinics of North America*, 30, March, 1–19.

Missmer, S.A., Hankinson, S.E., Spiegelman, D., et al. 2004. Incidence of Laparoscopically Confirmed Endometriosis by Demographic, Anthropometric, and Lifestyle Factors. *American Journal of Epidemiology*, 160(8), 784–96.

Moen, M.H. 1994. Endometriosis in monozygotic twins. *Acta Obstetricia et Gynecologica Scandinavica*, 73, 59–62.

Mol, A. 1999. Ontological politics. A word and some questions, in *Actor Network Theory and After,* edited by J. Law and J. Hassard. Oxford: Blackwell Publishers, 74–89.

Mol, A. 2002. *The Body Multiple: Ontology in Medical Practice.* Durham: Duke University Press.

Mol, A. and Law, J. 2002. Complexities: An introduction, in *Complexities: Social Studies of Knowledge Practices*, edited by J. Law and A. Mol. Durham: Duke University Press, 1–22.

Molgaard, C. and Gresham, L. 1985. Current concepts in endometriosis. *The Western Journal of Medicine*, 143(1), 42–6.

Mythen, G. 2004. *Ulrich Beck: A Critical Introduction to the Risk Society.* London: Pluto Press.

Nap, A. 2012. Theories on the pathogenesis of endometriosis, in *Endometriosis: Science and Practice*, edited by L. Giudice, J. Evers and D. Healy. Chichester: Wiley Blackwell, 42–53.

Nash, L. 2006. *Inescapable Ecologies: A History of Environment, Disease and Knowledge.* California: University of California Press.

Nettleton, S. 1995. *The Sociology of Health and Illness.* 1st Edition. Cambridge: Polity Press.

Nettleton, S. 1997. Governing the risky self: How to become healthy, wealthy and wise, in *Foucault Health and Medicine,* edited by A. Petersen and R. Bunton. London: Routledge, 207–22.

Nettleton, S. 2006. *The Sociology of Health and Illness.* 2nd Edition. Cambridge: Polity Press.

Newman, C., Bonar, M., Greville, H.S., et al. 2007. 'Everything is okay': The influence of neoliberal discourse on the reported experiences of Aboriginal people in Western Australia who are HIV-positive. *Culture, Health and Sexuality*, 9(6), 571–84.

Nezhat, C., King, L.P., Paka, C., et al. 2012. Bilateral thoracic endometriosis affecting the lung and diaphragm. *Journal of the Society of Endolaparoscopic Surgeons*, 16(1), 140–42.

Nezhat, C., Nezhat, F. and Nezhat. C. 2012. Endometriosis: Ancient disease, ancient treatments. *Fertility and Sterility*, 98(6 Supplement): S1–62.

Northrup, C. 1998. *Women's Bodies, Women's Wisdom: The Complete Guide to Women's Health and Wellbeing.* 2nd Edition. London: Judy Piatkus Publishers.

Norton, H. 2012. *Take Control of Your Endometriosis: Help Relieve Symptoms with Simple Diet and Lifestyle Changes.* London: Kyle Books.

Oakley, A. 1979. *From Here to Maternity: Becoming a Mother.* Harmondsworth: Penguin.

Oakley, A. 1981. Interviewing women: A contradiction in terms, in *Doing Feminist Research*, edited by H. Roberts. London: Routledge and Kegan Paul, 30–61.

Older, J. 1984. *Endometriosis*. New York: Charles Scribner's Sons.

Olive, D. and Pritts, E. 2001. Treatment of endometriosis. *The New England Journal of Medicine*, 345(4), 266–75.

Overton, C., Davis, C., McMillan, L. and Calman, J. 2002. *An Atlas of Endometriosis*. 2nd Edition. London: The Parthenon Publishing Group.

Oudshoorn, N. 1994. *Beyond the Natural Body: An Archeology of Sex Hormones*. London: Routledge.

Parazzini, F., Chiaffarino, F., Surace, M., et al. 2004. Selected food intake and risk of Endometriosis. *Human Reproduction*, 19(8), 1755–9.

Pauwels, A., Schepens, P.J.C., D'Hooghe, T., et al. 2001. The risk of endometriosis and exposure to dioxins and polychlorinated biphenyls: a case-control study of infertile women. *Human Reproduction*, 16(10), 2050–55.

Petersen, A. 1997a. The new morality: Public health and personal conduct, *Foucault: The Legacy*, edited by C. O'Farrell. Kelvin Grove: Queensland University of Technology, 696–706.

Petersen, A. 1997b. Risk, governance and the new public health, in *Foucault Health and Medicine*, edited by A. Petersen and R. Bunton. London: Routledge, 189–206.

Petersen, A. 2005. The metaphors of risk: biotechnology in the news. *Health, Risk and Society*, 7(3), 203–8.

Petersen, A. 2006. The best experts: The narratives of those who have a genetic condition, *Social Science and Medicine* 63(1), 32–4.

Petersen. A. and Wilkinson, I. 2008. Health, risk and vulnerability: an introduction, in *Health, Risk and Vulnerability*, edited by A. Petersen and I. Wilkinson. Abingdon: Routledge, 1–15.

Phillips, R.H and Motta, G. 2000. *Coping with Endometriosis*. New York: Avery.

Pinkert, T.C., Catlow, C. and Straus, R. 1979. Endometriosis of the urinary bladder in a man with prostatic carcinoma. *Cancer*, 43(4), 1562–7.

Pollock, G. 2003. Screening the seventies: Sexuality and representation in feminist practice – A Brechtian perspective, in *The Feminism and Visual Culture Reader*, edited by A. Jones. New York and London: Routledge, 76–93.

Possamai, A. 2000. A profile of new agers: social and spiritual aspects. *Journal of Sociology*, 36(3), 354–77.

Quinn, M. 2009. Endometriosis: The elusive epiphenomenon. *Journal of Obstetrics and Gynaecology*, 29(7), 590–93.

Redwine, D. 2002. Was Sampson wrong? *Fertility and Sterility*, 78(4), 686–93.

Redwine, D. 2003. 'Invisible' microscopic endometriosis: A Review. *Gynecologic and Obstetric Investigation*, 55: 63–7.

Redwine, D. 2009. *One Hundred Questions and Answers about Endometriosis*. Mississuaga: Jones and Bartlett Publishers.

Reger, J. 2001. Emotions, objectivity and voice: An analysis of a 'failed' participant observation. *Women's Studies International Forum*, 24(5): 605–16.

Rhodes, P. 1996. *Gynaecology for Everywoman.* Cheshire England: Haigh and Hochland Publications.

Rier, S. and Foster, W. 2002. Environmental toxins and endometriosis. *Toxicological Sciences*, 70, 161–70.

Rier, S., Martin, D.C., Bowman, R.E., et al. 1993. Endometriosis in rhesus monkeys (*Macaca Mulatta*) following chronic exposure to 2,3,7,8–Tetrachlorodibenzo-p–dioxin. *Fundamental and Applied Toxicology* 21, 433–41.

Rier, S., Turner, W.E., Martin, D.C., et al. 2001b. Serum levels of TCDD and Dioxin-like chemicals in rhesus monkeys chronically exposed to dioxin: Correlation of increased serum PCB levels with endometriosis. *Toxicological Sciences*, 59, 147–59.

Rier, S.E., Coe, C.L., Lemieux, A.M., Martin, D.C., et al. 2001a. Increased tumor necrosis factor–a production by peripheral blood leukocytes from TCDD-exposed rhesus monkeys. *Toxicological Sciences*, 60, 327–37.

Riessman, C.K. 2002. Analysis of personal narratives, in *Handbook of Interview Research: Context and Method*, edited by J.F. Gubrium and J.A. Holstein. Thousand Oaks: California: Sage, 695–710.

Rimke, H. 2000. Governing citizens through self-help literature. *Cultural Studies*, 14(1), 61–78.

Roberts, C. 2007. *Messengers of Sex: Hormones, Biomedicine and Feminism.* New York: Cambridge University Press.

Robertson, A. 2000. Embodying risk, embodying political rationality: women's accounts of risks for breast cancer. *Health Risk and Society*, 2(2), 219–35.

Robertson, A. 2001. Biotechnology, political rationality and discourses on health risk. *Health: An Interdisciplinary Journal for the Social Study of Health, Illness and Medicine*, 5(3), 293–309.

von Rokitansky, C. 1860. Ueber uterusdrusden-neubildung im uterus and ovariansarcomen. *Zkk Gesellsch D Aertze Zu Wein*; 37, 577.

Rose, G. 2005. What is endometriosis? *Women's Health Medicine*, 2(1), 12–14.

Rose, N. 1996. *Inventing Our Selves: Psychology, Power, and Personhood.* Cambridge: Cambridge University Press.

Rose, N. 1999. *Governing the Soul: The Shaping of the Private Self.* 2nd Edition. London: Free Association Books.

Rose, N. 2007. *The Politics of Life Itself.* Princeton: Princeton University Press.

Royal College of Obstetricians and Gynaecologists 2006. The investigation and management of endometriosis. *Green-Top Guideline*, 24, 1–14.

Saldanha, A. 2003. Actor-Network theory and critical sociology. *Critical Sociology*, 29(3), 419–32.

Sampson, J.A. 1921. Perforating hemorrhagic (chocolate) cysts of the ovary. *Arch. Surg.*, 3, 245–53.

Sampson, J.A. 1925a. Inguinal endometriosis (often reported as endometrial t in the groin, adenomyoma in the groin, and adenomyoma of the round ligament. *American Journal of Obstetrics and Gynecology*, 10, 462–503.

Sampson, J.A. 1925b. Heterotopic or misplaced endometrial tissue. *American Journal of Obstetrics and Gynecology*, 10, 649–64.

Sarma, D., Iyengar, P., Marotta, T.R., et al. 2004. Cerebellar endometriosis. *American Journal of Roentgenology*, 182(6): 1543–6.

Scott, R. and TeLinde, R. 1950. External endometriosis – The scourge of the private patient. *Annals of Surgery*, 131(5), 697–719.

Seear, K. 2004. *The Hidden Body.* Unpublished Honours Dissertation. Clayton: Monash University.

Seear, K. 2009a. 'Standing up to the beast': Contradictory notions of control, un/certainty and risk in the endometriosis self-help literature. *Critical Public Health*, 19(1), 45–58.

Seear, K. 2009b. The third shift: Health, work and expertise among women with endometriosis. *Health Sociology Review*, 18(2), 194–206.

Seear, K. 2009c. The etiquette of endometriosis: Stigmatisation, menstrual concealment and the diagnostic delay. *Social Science & Medicine*, 69, 1220–27.

Seear, K. 2009d. 'Nobody really knows what it is or how to treat it': Why women with endometriosis do not comply with healthcare advice. *Health, Risk and Society*, 11(4), 367–85.

Seear, K. and Fraser, S. 2010a. 'The sorry addict': Ben Cousins and the construction of drug use in elite sport. *Health Sociology Review*, 19(2), 176–91.

Seear, K. and Fraser, S. 2010b. Ben Cousins and the 'double life': Exploring citizenship and the voluntarity/compulsivity binary through the experiences of a 'drug addicted' elite athlete. *Critical Public Health*, 20(4), 439–52.

Seear, K., Fraser, S. and Lenton, E. 2010. Guilty or angry? The politics of emotion in accounts of hepatitis C transmission. *Contemporary Drug Problems*, 37(4), 619–38.

Shildrick, M. 1997. *Leaky Bodies and Boundaries: Feminism, Postmodernism and (Bio)Ethics*. London: Routledge.

Shohat, E. 1998. 'Lasers for Ladies': Endo Discourse and the inscriptions of science, in *The Visible Woman: Imaging Technologies, Gender and Science*, edited by P.A. Treichler, L. Cartwright and C. Penley. New York: New York University Press, 240–70.

Signorile, P. and Baldi, A. 2010. Endometriosis: New concepts in the pathogenesis. *The International Journal of Biochemistry and Cell Biology*, 42, 778–80.

Simeons, S., Hummelshoj, L. and D'Hooghe, T. 2007. Endometriosis: Cost estimates and methodological perspective. *Human Reproduction*, 13(4), 395–404.

Simeons, S., Dunselman, G., Dirksen, C., et al, T. 2012. The burden of endometriosis: costs and quality of life of women with endometriosis and treated in referral centres. *Human Reproduction*, 21(5), 1292–9.

Simonds, W. 1992. *Women and Self-Help Culture: Reading between the Lines*. New Brunswick: Rutgers University Press.

Simonds, W. 1996. All consuming selves: self-help literature and women's identities, in *Constructing the Self in a Mediated World*, edited by D. Grodin and T.R. Lindlof. Thousand Oaks, CA: Sage, 15–29.

Singer, L. 1993. *Erotic Welfare: Sexual Theory and Politics in the Age of Epidemic*, New York and London: Routledge.

Singleton, A. 2003. 'Men's bodies, men's selves': Men's health self-help books and the promotion of health care. *International Journal of Men's Health*, 2(1), 57–72.

Singleton, A. 2004. Good advice for Godly men: Oppressed men in Christian men's self-help literature. *Journal of Gender Studies*, 13(2), 153–64.

Sloan, W. 1947. The problem of endometriosis; a review. *The Ulster Medical Journal*, 16(1), 27–32.

Slovic, P. 1986. Informing and educating the public about risk. *Risk Analysis*, 6(4), 403–15.

Sontag, S. 2001. *Illness as Metaphor and AIDS and Its Metaphors*. New York: Picador.

Stacey, J. 1997. *Teratologies: A Cultural Study of Cancer.* London: Routledge.

Starker, S. 1989. *Oracle at the Supermarket*. New Brunswick: Transaction Publishers.

Steptoe, P. 1967. *Laparoscopy in Gynaecology*. Edinburgh, Livingstone.

Stratton, P. 2006. The tangled web of reasons for the delay in diagnosis of endometriosis in women with chronic pelvic pain: will the suffering end? *Fertility and Sterility*, 86(5), 1302–4.

Strzempko Butt, F. and Chesla, C. 2007. Relational patterns of couples living with chronic pelvic pain from endometriosis. *Qualitative Health Research*, 17(5), 571–85.

Surrey, E.S. and Hornstein, M.D. 2002. Prolonged GnRH agonist and add-back therapy for symptomatic endometriosis: Long-term follow-up. *Obstetrics and Gynecology*, 99(5), Part 1, 709–19.

Sutton, C. and Jones, K. 2004. *Endometriosis*. London: Royal College of Obstetricians and Gynaecologists Press.

TeLinde, R.W. and Mattingly, R.F. 1970. *Operative Gynecology*. 4th Edition. Philadelphia: Lippincott.

Thomas, E.J. 1993. Endometriosis: still an enigma. *British Journal of Obstetrics and Gynaecology*, 100, 615–17.

Treichler, P. 1999. *How to Have Theory in an Epidemic: Cultural Chronicles of AIDS*. Durham: Duke University Press.

Treloar, S.A., Wicks, J., Nyholt, D.R., et al. 2005. Genomewide linkage study in 1,176 affected sister pair families identifies a significant susceptibility locus for endometriosis on chromosome 10q26. *American Journal of Human Genetics*, 77, 365–76.

Ussher, J. 2003. Biology as Destiny: The legacy of Victorian gynaecology in the 21st century. *Feminism and Psychology*, 13(1), 17–22.

Ussher, J. 2006. Managing the Monstrous Feminine: Regulating the Reproductive Body. East Sussex: Routledge.

Vanden Heuvel, J.P., Clark, G.C., Tritscher, A.M. and Lucier, G.W. 1994. Accumulation of polychlorinated dibenzo-*P*-dioxins and dibenzofurans in liver of control laboratory rats. *Fundamental and Applied Toxicology*, 23, 465–69.

Vanderhaege, L. 2000. Endometriosis epidemic. *Total Health*, 22(6), 34–6.

Varma, R., Rollason, T., Gupta, J. and Maher, E. 2004. Endometriosis and the neoplastic process. *Reproduction*, 127, 293–304.

Vitellone, N. 2011. The science of the syringe. *Feminist Theory*. 12(2), 201–7.

Waldby, C. 1996. *AIDS and the Body Politic: Biomedicine and Sexual Difference*. London: Routledge.

Wang, G., Tokushige, N., Markham, R. and Fraser, I.S. 2009. Rich innervation of deep infiltrating endometriosis. *Human Reproduction*, .24(4), 827–34.

Way, S. 1964. Obituaries: Joe Vincent Meigs. *Journal of Obstetrics and Gynaecology*, 310–12.

Weinstein, K. 1987. *Living with Endometriosis: How to Cope with the Physical and Emotional Challenges*. Massachusetts, USA: Addison-Wesley Publishing Company.

Weir, E. 2001. The public health toll of endometriosis. *Canadian Medical Association Journal*, 164(8), 1201.

Whelan, E. 1997. Staging and profiling: The constitution of the endometriotic subject in gynecological discourse. *Alternate Routes*, 14, 45–68.

Whelan, E. 2000. *Well Now, Who's the Doctor Here? Boundary-Work and Transgression in Lay and Expert Knowledges of Endometriosis*. Unpublished PhD dissertation. Ottawa, Canada: Carleton University.

Whelan, E. 2003. Putting pain to paper: endometriosis and the documentation of suffering. *Health*, 7(4), 463–82.

Whelan, E. 2007. 'No one agrees except for those of us who have it': endometriosis patients as an epistemological community. *Sociology of Health and Illness*, 29(7), 1–26.

Wren, B. 1979. *Handbook of Obstetrics and Gynaecology*. New South Wales: Cassell Australia Limited.

Wright, J. and Shafik, A. 2001. Quality of life following excision of rectovaginal endometriosis associated with complete obliteration of the posterior cul de sac. *Gynaecol Endosc* 10, 107–11.

Yu, J.H., Lin, X.Y., Wang, L., et al. 2013. Endobronchial endometriosis presenting as central-type lung cancer: a case report. *Diagnostic Pathology*, 8, 53.

Zeyneloglu, H., Arici, A. and Olive, D. 1997. Environmental toxins and endometriosis. *Obstetrics and Gynecology Clinics*, 24(2), 307–29.

Zola, I.K. 1972. Medicine as an institution of social control. *Sociological Review*, 20, 487–504.

Index

Milton Keynes UK
Ingram Content Group UK Ltd.
UKHW040057071024
449327UK00019B/618